Anya Celeste

Ho'oponopono Essential
Caring for the Mind and Soul

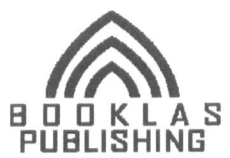

Original Title: Ho'oponopono Essencial
Copyright © 2025, published by Luiz Antonio dos Santos ME.

This book is a work of non-fiction that explores practices and concepts in the field of personal development and abundance. Through a comprehensive approach, the author offers practical tools to achieve emotional balance, prosperity, and personal fulfillment.

**1st Edition**
**Production Team**
**Author:** Anya Celeste
**Editor:** Luiz Santos
**Cover:** Studios Booklas / Guilhermo Anturus
**Layout:** Zara Cruz
**Translation:** Mark Bennet

Publication and Identification Ho'oponopono Essential Booklas, 2025
Categories: Personal Development / Spirituality / Holism DDC: 158.1 - CDU: 159.923.2

All rights reserved to:
Luiz Antonio dos Santos ME / Booklas
No part of this book may be reproduced, stored in a retrieval system, or transmitted by any means - electronic, mechanical, photocopying, recording, or otherwise - without [1] the prior and express permission of the copyright [2] holder.

# Summary

Prologue .................................................................................. 5
Chapter 1 Understanding Ho'oponopono .......................... 7
Chapter 2 Inner Cleansing................................................. 14
Chapter 3 The Essence of Healing .................................... 21
Chapter 4 The Mantra of Healing ..................................... 28
Chapter 5 Manifesting Your Desires ................................. 35
Chapter 6 Anchoring in the Present .................................. 42
Chapter 7 Deepening the Connection ............................... 50
Chapter 8 Harmony in Bonds............................................ 58
Chapter 9 Healing the Roots ............................................. 65
Chapter 10 Freeing Yourself from the Chains .................. 72
Chapter 11 Self-Esteem .................................................... 79
Chapter 12 Abundant Prosperity....................................... 87
Chapter 13 Inner Harmony, Healthy Body ....................... 94
Chapter 14 Inner Flow ...................................................... 101
Chapter 15 Legacies of the Past........................................ 108
Chapter 16 Ho'oponopono for Children............................ 115
Chapter 17 Harmony and Healing in the Relationship ..... 122
Chapter 18 Financial Prosperity with Awareness ............. 129
Chapter 19 Home Purification .......................................... 136
Chapter 20 Messages from the Subconscious................... 143
Chapter 21 Aging with Wisdom and Serenity .................. 150
Chapter 22 Finding Relief and Healing ............................ 157
Chapter 23 Transforming the Energy of Fire.................... 164
Chapter 24 Releasing Fear ................................................ 171

Chapter 25 Anxiety: Calming the Mind .................................... 178
Chapter 26 Depression, Self-Healing and Hope ...................... 185
Chapter 27 Consolation in the Pain of Loss ............................. 193
Chapter 28 Freeing Yourself from the Bonds of the Past ......... 200
Chapter 29 Connecting with the Divine Essence ..................... 207
Chapter 30 Energetic Harmony ................................................ 214
Chapter 31 Healing with the Power of Sound .......................... 222
Chapter 32 Law of Attraction ................................................... 229
Chapter 33 Advanced Ho'oponopono ....................................... 236
Chapter 34 Inspiring Transformation ........................................ 243
Epilogue ..................................................................................... 250

# Prologue

It is with immense satisfaction that I place in your hands this book that carries not just words, but an ancestral wisdom capable of transforming lives. Ho'oponopono is not just a practice; it is a silent and profound invitation to revisit one's own essence, heal memories, dissolve blockages, and rescue inner balance.

Upon encountering this work, I was touched by the simplicity and depth of its teachings. In a world so accelerated and full of noise, finding a path that returns us to inner peace is a rare gift. Each page you are about to explore reveals a practical and accessible philosophy, based on four powerful phrases: "I'm sorry. Please forgive me. I love you. I'm grateful." These words carry a transformative force capable of healing invisible pains and restoring lost connections - with others, with the world, and especially with yourself.

This book does not offer ready-made formulas, but a sincere invitation to self-responsibility and unconditional love. It is a guide for those seeking answers and, even more so, for those who are ready to ask the right questions.

Allow yourself to immerse yourself in this reading with an open heart. With each chapter, you will realize that true transformation begins from the inside out. The path may be silent, but the results echo deeply in the soul.

May this work inspire you to release what no longer serves, to forgive with lightness, to love without reservation, and to be grateful for every step of this journey.

Good reading and a profound journey of healing,
Luiz Santos Editor

# Chapter 1
# Understanding Ho'oponopono

Ho'oponopono is revealed as a transformative practice, based on ancient Hawaiian wisdom, that guides individuals to achieve emotional, mental, and spiritual balance through self-awareness and personal responsibility. This philosophy of life invites deep reflection on one's own thoughts, memories, and beliefs, highlighting the importance of recognizing that all lived experiences are internal reflections that can be understood and reframed. By applying its principles, such as forgiveness, repentance, gratitude, and unconditional love, it is possible to promote inner reconciliation and harmony in interpersonal relationships, leading to a journey of continuous healing and expansion of consciousness. This practical and accessible approach allows anyone to initiate a process of self-transformation, dissolving emotional blocks and releasing limiting patterns that impede the natural flow of life.

The practice of Ho'oponopono stimulates connection with the inner essence, recognizing that change begins with the acknowledgment of individual responsibilities. Through simple repetitions of powerful phrases, such as "I'm sorry," "Please forgive me," "I love you," and "I'm grateful," the individual activates a process of cleansing subconscious memories that generate conflicts and imbalances. This method does not require complex rituals or intermediaries, making it an effective tool for those seeking to transform daily challenges into opportunities for growth. This simplicity, combined with the depth of its results, allows Ho'oponopono to fit naturally into various cultures and lifestyles, consolidating itself as an accessible path to integral well-being.

By integrating Ho'oponopono into everyday life, a space of self-compassion and acceptance is created, where the past ceases to be a burden and becomes understood as part of the evolutionary journey. This continuous practice facilitates the detachment from resentments, fears, and limitations, allowing energy to flow lightly and in a balanced way. By taking full responsibility for everything that manifests, one opens the possibility of cultivating more harmonious relationships, strengthening emotional and mental health, and boosting personal and spiritual fulfillment. Ho'oponopono, therefore, not only heals but also guides the construction of a life based on peace, love, and true inner freedom.

The word "Ho'oponopono" carries within itself a profound essence of Hawaiian culture, translating as "to correct an error" or "to make right." This expression reveals more than just a linguistic concept; it represents a philosophy of life aimed at restoring balance and harmony. In Hawaiian tradition, Ho'oponopono was widely used as a collective healing ritual, applied within families and communities to resolve conflicts, restore relationships, and rebalance vital energy. There was a belief that physical and emotional illnesses arose as reflections of internal imbalances and disharmony in interpersonal relationships. Thus, Ho'oponopono emerged as a way to clear these blockages and allow energy to flow freely again.

In traditional gatherings, the process was led by a kahuna, a highly respected figure recognized as a priest or healer. This spiritual leader guided participants through prayers, sincere confessions, and purification rituals. Each member involved was encouraged to acknowledge their mistakes, express remorse, and ask for forgiveness, thus promoting a deep cleansing not only of emotions but also of the energies that sustained the conflicts. Reconciliation was not only desirable but essential, as it was believed that individual healing contributed directly to the health and balance of the entire community. The interconnection between individuals was seen as something sacred and inseparable, and the harmony of one reflected in the well-being of all.

Over the centuries, Ho'oponopono has not remained static. It has adapted to social and cultural changes, expanding its application beyond Hawaiian communities. This evolution was profoundly influenced by Morrnah Nalamaku Simeona, a respected kahuna who, in the 20th century, reformulated the practice to make it more accessible to the modern world. Morrnah realized that for Ho'oponopono to reach a wider audience, it would be necessary to adapt its rituals without losing its essence. Thus, she developed an individualized approach, allowing anyone to apply the principles of Ho'oponopono autonomously, without the need for a spiritual leader. This transformation made the practice simpler and applicable to everyday life, regardless of religious or cultural beliefs.

In the modern version of Ho'oponopono, the emphasis is on personal responsibility. According to this perspective, everything we experience in our external reality is a direct reflection of memories and beliefs stored in our subconscious. These memories, often invisible to consciousness, shape our perceptions, reactions, and experiences. By turning inward and recognizing that we are co-creators of our own reality, we can initiate a profound process of cleansing and transformation. This purification happens through the repetition of simple but powerful phrases: "I'm sorry," "Please forgive me," "I love you," and "I'm grateful." Each word carries a specific intention that acts directly on the release of negative memories and patterns, allowing peace and clarity to return to our being.

The fundamental principles of Ho'oponopono underpin this practice with solidity. Full responsibility is the foundation, as it implies accepting that everything that happens in our life is, in some way, connected to us. This does not mean guilt, but rather power — the power to transform what no longer serves us. Interconnection reinforces the idea that our actions, thoughts, and emotions influence not only ourselves but also the entire environment around us. Forgiveness emerges as a healing balm, releasing deep hurts and dissolving emotional barriers. Repentance, in turn, is a gesture of humility that acknowledges faults and opens space for reconciliation. Gratitude elevates the inner vibration, directing focus to the blessings present, while unconditional love permeates the entire practice, being the most powerful force of healing and transformation.

The benefits of Ho'oponopono are vast and encompass various spheres of life. By clearing negative memories, one experiences genuine inner peace, a serenity that does not depend on external circumstances. Relationships are also positively impacted, as the practice dissolves resentments and facilitates sincere dialogue, creating stronger and more harmonious bonds. Physical and emotional health tends to improve, as the release of internal tensions directly reflects on the body and mind. Furthermore, by eliminating limiting beliefs related to prosperity, a path is opened to a more abundant life in all aspects. Self-knowledge is inevitable in this process, as Ho'oponopono leads to an inner journey of discovery and recognition of one's true essence. This path, finally, leads to spiritual growth, connecting the individual with their inner divinity and expanding their consciousness.

This deep integration of Ho'oponopono into everyday life transforms challenges into opportunities for growth. The continuous practice of these simple but powerful words acts as a constant reminder that we are responsible for our own reality and that we have the power to change any situation. With each repetition, a silent and effective cleansing takes place, dissolving painful memories and opening space for new experiences. Thus, Ho'oponopono becomes a living practice, accompanying the flow of life, adapting to the needs of each moment. It invites self-compassion, forgiveness, and gratitude, creating a solid foundation for a lighter, more fluid, and meaningful existence.

With this understanding, it is clear that Ho'oponopono is not just a healing technique, but a philosophy of life that guides human beings to live in harmony with themselves and with the world. It teaches us that true transformation begins from the inside out and that by healing our own pain, we contribute to collective healing. This ancestral practice, even adapted to the modern context, maintains its essence intact: the search for peace, reconciliation, and unconditional love. Thus, Ho'oponopono continues to be a bridge between the past and the present, between the inner self and the universe around, guiding each individual to a state of greater balance, understanding, and fulfillment.

The Path of Healing: When walking the path of healing through Ho'oponopono, each step taken represents a return to one's own center, where authenticity and peace are found. This continuous process does not require perfection, but rather presence and willingness to recognize and release patterns that no longer serve us. The constant practice of sacred phrases functions as a gentle invitation to revisit our deepest emotions and, with kindness, dissolve blocks that obscure our well-being. Thus, healing happens naturally and progressively, guiding the practitioner to a state of greater clarity and lightness in everyday life.

By appropriating this ancestral knowledge, we begin to realize that true transformation is not about changing the external world, but about adjusting our perception and our inner vibration. This subtle change reverberates in all areas of life, positively influencing our thoughts, attitudes, and relationships. Ho'oponopono then becomes a bridge between self-knowledge and full realization, allowing each challenge faced to be seen as an opportunity for learning and evolution.

In this way, Ho'oponopono is revealed not only as a spiritual practice, but as a daily invitation to live with more awareness, compassion, and love. By integrating its principles into everyday life, we open space for a more harmonious and true existence, where inner peace ceases to be a distant ideal and becomes a tangible reality. Thus, a continuous journey of healing and growth begins, guided by the wisdom that we are fully responsible for creating the life we wish to live.

# Chapter 2
# Inner Cleansing

True personal transformation begins with the decision to free oneself from memories and beliefs that limit growth and happiness. This process involves a deep purification of the subconscious, where past experiences, repressed emotions, and behavior patterns are stored, directly influencing how we live and relate to others. By taking responsibility for these memories, it becomes possible to dissolve inner blockages, promoting emotional and mental healing. This path of self-knowledge and inner renewal opens space for the true self to flourish, bringing lightness, clarity, and balance to life. Inner cleansing, therefore, is not just an abstract concept, but a constant practice of self-understanding and self-love, capable of transforming the way we perceive the world and how we interact with it.

The Subconscious: An Ocean of Memories

Imagine our subconscious as a vast ocean, full of memories, beliefs, and emotions that accumulate throughout life. Every experience, every interaction, every thought leaves a mark on this inner ocean. Many of these memories are positive and propel us towards growth, but we also carry with us painful memories, traumas, and limiting beliefs that act as anchors, preventing us from achieving fullness and happiness.

These negative memories manifest themselves in our lives in various ways: repetitive behavior patterns, dysfunctional relationships, creative blocks, health problems, scarcity, and difficulties in manifesting our dreams. As long as these memories remain in our subconscious, they will continue to influence our choices and shape our reality.

Identifying the memories and beliefs that generate disharmony in life is an essential step to begin the process of inner cleansing. Often, these limiting patterns are so ingrained that they go unnoticed, influencing thoughts, emotions, and behaviors in subtle yet constant ways. Self-awareness, therefore, becomes a fundamental tool on this journey. Carefully observing one's own reactions to challenging situations can reveal the deep roots of emotional blocks. When recurring feelings of anger, fear, sadness, or frustration emerge, it is a sign that there are old memories asking to be recognized and released.

This identification process requires courage and compassion. Questioning oneself deeply - "Why do I always feel this way?", "What is really stopping me from moving forward?" or "What beliefs sustain my limitations?" - opens space for valuable insights. It is important to embrace each answer without judgment, understanding that carrying these memories is part of the human experience. Self-criticism does not contribute to healing; on the contrary, it can reinforce patterns of suffering. True transformation happens when you look inward with kindness, recognizing that each challenge carries within it an opportunity for growth.

To assist in this journey of self-knowledge and liberation, Ho'oponopono offers simple but profoundly effective tools. The four sacred phrases - "I'm sorry. Please forgive me. I love you. Thank you." - are the foundation of this practice. By pronouncing them sincerely, a cleansing process begins that goes beyond words, touching the deepest layers of the subconscious. These phrases function as keys that unlock inner doors, allowing painful memories to be recognized, accepted, and finally dissolved. Each word carries a specific vibration: repentance acknowledges the impact of memories, the request for forgiveness releases guilt, love heals, and gratitude consolidates transformation.

Visualization also presents itself as a powerful tool in the cleansing process. Imagining negative memories as dark clouds slowly dissipating in the blue sky or as heavy stones being gently carried away by the current of a river brings a sense of relief and lightness. These mental images help in deconstructing ingrained patterns, allowing the mind and heart to open to new possibilities. Conscious breathing complements this process. By inhaling deeply, the body is oxygenated and the mind is cleared; by exhaling slowly, accumulated tension and stagnant energies are released. This calm rhythm of breathing serves as an invitation to relaxation and detachment from thoughts that no longer serve.

The process of inner cleansing occurs in delicate and interconnected stages. First, it is necessary to bring to consciousness the memory or belief that you want to transform. It is not about reliving the pain, but about recognizing it as part of the journey that needs to be understood and released. By taking responsibility for this memory, it is understood that, regardless of how or when it arose, it is now part of the internal universe, and it is possible to heal it. Then, the repetition of the Ho'oponopono phrases should be done with surrender and truth, directing this healing energy to the memory in question. At the same time, visualization helps to materialize this release process, and conscious breathing leads to the relaxation necessary for the transformation to occur naturally.

Trusting the process is essential. The mind often seeks immediate results, but inner cleansing follows the proper flow of time and the depth of each experience. Having faith in the inner divinity and the power of personal healing strengthens this path. Each practice, however simple it may seem, contributes to dissolving layers of resistance and opening space for a new way of being. This commitment to self-healing, repeated day after day, generates subtle changes that, over time, are reflected in major transformations.

With the continuity of this practice, the effects begin to manifest in a perceptible way. Relationships previously marked by tension become lighter and more harmonious. Decisions are made with more clarity, without the interference of fears or insecurities. Obstacles that seemed insurmountable are faced with serenity, and often dissolve naturally. This process is not abrupt, but fluid and constant, the result of genuine dedication to self-knowledge and the release of old patterns. The emotional burden of the past gradually dissolves, giving way to a growing sense of freedom and authenticity.

As the mind is purified, the connection with intuition is strengthened. The inner voice becomes clearer, guiding decisions more aligned with the true essence. This inner balance allows us to see challenges from a new perspective, recognizing them as opportunities for evolution. The peace that arises from this process is solid and consistent, based on the awareness that each individual is responsible for co-creating their own reality. This state of serenity does not depend on external circumstances, but on the harmony cultivated internally.

This journey of inner cleansing is not only a path of healing, but also of personal expansion. By freeing ourselves from limiting memories, we create space for the emergence of new possibilities. Self-love is strengthened, gratitude becomes a natural state, and compassion for oneself and others flourishes. This reunion with the purest essence of being brings with it the wisdom, peace, and strength necessary to live authentically. Each step on this journey is an invitation to be more present, lighter, and truer to oneself and to the world.

Thus, the continuous practice of inner cleansing through Ho'oponopono is revealed as a safe and profound path of self-transformation. It is a process that requires surrender, patience, and above all, love. By recognizing, accepting, and releasing what limits us, we open space for a fuller life, where inner peace is not a distant ideal, but a tangible reality. In this constant flow of healing and growth, each challenge faced becomes a new opportunity for evolution, gently guiding us to a state of balance, harmony, and fulfillment.

Over time, the constant practice of these inner cleansing tools begins to reflect in perceptible changes in everyday life. Relationships previously marked by conflict become more harmonious, decisions are made with more clarity and confidence, and challenges that seemed insurmountable begin to be overcome with lightness. This transformation does not occur abruptly, but as a natural flow, a result of daily commitment to self-knowledge and the release of old patterns. The weight of past experiences is being replaced by a growing sense of freedom and authenticity.

As the mind is purified, the connection with intuition is strengthened, guiding choices more aligned with the true essence. This state of inner balance allows us to see life with new eyes, where each challenge becomes an opportunity for growth and learning. The peace that emerges from this process is not fragile or fleeting, but deep and consistent, sustained by the awareness that we are co-creators of our reality. Thus, the journey of inner cleansing is revealed as a continuous path of personal expansion and evolution.

Cultivating this inner space of serenity and clarity opens doors to a fuller and more meaningful existence. When we free ourselves from the shackles of the past, we create space for new experiences and possibilities, allowing self-love, gratitude, and compassion to flourish naturally. This is the true purpose of inner cleansing: to provide a reunion with the purest essence of being, where the wisdom, peace, and strength necessary to live authentically reside. Thus, each step on this journey becomes an invitation to live with more presence, lightness, and truth.

# Chapter 3
# The Essence of Healing

Unconditional Love represents the purest and most transformative force capable of promoting true inner healing. It is born from the total acceptance of who we are and extends unreservedly to all beings, without judgments or conditions. This loving energy transcends limitations, dissolving emotional and mental barriers that impede the natural flow of harmony and peace. When we embrace this form of love, we allow feelings of forgiveness, compassion, and gratitude to flow freely, creating space for reconciliation with ourselves and with the world around us. This love is the maximum expression of our divine essence, a direct connection with the creative source, which drives us to live with more lightness, understanding, and balance.

By allowing Unconditional Love to guide our thoughts and actions, we pave the way for a profound transformation. It invites us to look at our own imperfections with kindness, recognizing that our mistakes and challenges are part of the journey of evolution. This love also teaches us to see the other with empathy, understanding that everyone carries stories and scars that influence their attitudes. With this, we learn to release resentments and judgments, replacing them with acceptance and compassion. This internal movement creates a solid foundation for true forgiveness, where emotional healing becomes possible and relationships are strengthened by mutual understanding.

Living Unconditional Love daily is a commitment to self-care and the expansion of consciousness. By nurturing this love within us, we cultivate a lighter and healthier internal environment, reflecting this positive energy in our relationships and in the environment around us. This continuous practice expands our capacity to love, strengthens our connection with the universe, and makes us instruments of healing and transformation. Thus, Unconditional Love not only restores our own essence but also inspires positive changes in the world, promoting peace, unity, and collective balance.

The love that transcends limitations is the essence of true healing. This unconditional love does not impose conditions, does not judge, and expects nothing in return. It simply is. It is born from the recognition of one's own inner divinity and extends to all beings, dissolving barriers built by the ego and the painful experiences of the past. This pure and absolute love does not distinguish between mistakes or successes but welcomes everything as part of the evolutionary process. In the context of Ho'oponopono, unconditional love is the foundation that sustains the practice, being the silent force that drives emotional, mental, and spiritual healing. It is through this love that we open ourselves to forgiveness, recognizing that both our faults and those of others are part of a greater path of learning.

Practicing Ho'oponopono with unconditional love means going beyond the desire to alleviate momentary suffering. It means involving painful memories with understanding and tenderness, without resistance or judgment. Instead of harboring resentment or guilt, we choose to direct love to the parts of ourselves that are still wounded. This simple but powerful gesture initiates a profound transformation, as each memory stored in our subconscious is gently enveloped by this healing energy. We recognize that even the most painful memories have a purpose and that they deserve to be looked at with compassion, and then released.

This practice teaches us that we are all in constant evolution, carrying stories and wounds that shape our actions. Unconditional love allows us to see the other with empathy, understanding that each person acts according to the emotional baggage they carry. Thus, there is no longer room for judgments or criticism, only for full acceptance. This acceptance creates an environment conducive to true forgiveness, not the one that seeks to justify or forget, but the one that understands and liberates. This internal movement not only relieves pain but also strengthens relationships, creating bonds based on mutual understanding and respect.

However, for us to offer this love to the world, it must first flourish within us. Self-love is the first step on this journey. To love oneself unconditionally implies accepting every part of oneself, including flaws, weaknesses, and moments of vulnerability. It means forgiving yourself for mistakes made and welcoming yourself with kindness. This self-love is not an act of selfishness but an expression of respect and care for one's own existence. It is understanding that by taking care of yourself with affection, you create a solid foundation for loving others genuinely.

To cultivate this unconditional love, some practices can be incorporated into everyday life. Self-knowledge is fundamental. Taking time to reflect on one's own thoughts, emotions, and behaviors allows one to identify beliefs and patterns that need to be reframed. This process requires sincerity and willingness to face internal aspects that we often prefer to avoid. Forgiveness, both of oneself and others, is another essential practice. Releasing hurts and resentments opens space for love to flow more lightly. Compassion also plays a central role, as it recognizes that everyone faces challenges and that pain is a universal experience.

Gratitude is another powerful way to strengthen unconditional love. By giving thanks for experiences, even those that have brought pain, we recognize that everything contributes to our growth. This positive attitude transforms the way we perceive life and deepens our connection with the present. Meditation, in turn, silences the mind and allows us to connect with the heart, where pure love resides. Positive affirmations are also effective tools, as they reprogram the mind to recognize self-worth and connection to the divine essence. Phrases like "I love and accept myself fully" or "I am worthy of love and happiness" reinforce this loving vibration.

Unconditional love, when cultivated, has a transformative power that goes beyond the individual. It expands naturally, reaching those around us and creating waves of healing and harmony. Small gestures of kindness, understanding, and empathy become seeds of transformation. When we choose to act with love, we contribute to a more peaceful and compassionate environment. Every loving attitude reverberates, creating a positive impact that extends beyond our personal relationships and influences the collective.

This deep understanding that we are all interconnected leads us to value our daily choices. We begin to act with more emotional responsibility, recognizing that our thoughts, words, and actions have the power to build or destroy. Respect for differences, attentive listening, and willingness to help others become natural expressions of this limitless love. Thus, the practice of unconditional love calls us to action, inviting us to be agents of peace and transformation in the world.

This loving energy, when fully experienced, reminds us that healing the other is also healing ourselves. The pain we recognize in the other often reflects wounds that have not yet been healed within us. By offering understanding and affection to others, we also soften our own pain. This continuous cycle of giving and receiving love strengthens the feeling of unity, dissolving the illusion of separation. We realize, then, that the path to collective healing begins with our own willingness to love without conditions.

Thus, unconditional love is revealed as a daily invitation to live with more truth and presence. By choosing to love without reservation, we embrace all of life's experiences, recognizing that each challenge brings with it an opportunity for learning and growth. This love transforms pain into wisdom, brings hearts closer, and illuminates paths. It reminds us that we are part of something greater and that, by cultivating it within us, we contribute to a more just, harmonious, and compassionate world.

Following this path is allowing yourself to be led by a subtle and powerful force, capable of dissolving internal and external barriers. It is trusting that, by living guided by love, we are always on the right path. This choice leads us to a lighter, more authentic, and fuller existence, where each step is permeated by peace and a deep connection with all that exists. Thus, unconditional love becomes not just a practice, but a way of being, a natural state that transforms lives and inspires the construction of a more loving and balanced world.

This loving energy expands naturally, reaching those with whom we live and inspiring subtle but profound changes. Small gestures of understanding and empathy become seeds of transformation, capable of softening conflicts and strengthening bonds. As we become channels of this healing force, we realize that every loving attitude reverberates beyond us, creating waves of balance and serenity that touch the collective. Thus, Unconditional Love ceases to be just an individual practice and is transformed into a silent movement of healing that crosses borders and connects hearts.

By understanding that we are all interconnected by this same essence, we begin to value the importance of our daily choices. Respect for differences, attentive listening, and willingness to help become natural expressions of this love that knows no bounds. This awareness awakens in us the responsibility to act with more kindness and compassion, recognizing that every positive gesture contributes to a more just and harmonious world. On this path, we realize that healing the other is also a way of healing ourselves.

In this way, cultivating Unconditional Love is more than an exercise in self-knowledge; it is an invitation to live more fully and truthfully. When we choose to love without condition, we embrace the totality of the human experience and align ourselves with universal wisdom. This love transforms pain into learning, strengthens relationships, and illuminates the path to a lighter and more authentic existence. Thus, we move forward, allowing this subtle and powerful force to lead us, step by step, towards a life of healing, peace, and deep connection with all that exists.

# Chapter 4
## The Mantra of Healing

The four phrases of Ho'oponopono — "I'm sorry. Please forgive me. I love you. I'm grateful." — represent a powerful synthesis of healing and personal transformation. Each word carries a unique vibration that acts directly on the subconscious, promoting the cleansing of memories and limiting patterns that shape our reality. This mantra is not just a sequence of words, but a profound invitation to self-responsibility, forgiveness, unconditional love, and gratitude. When expressed sincerely, these phrases trigger a process of inner purification, allowing reconciliation with ourselves and with the world around us. This continuous flow of recognition, release, love, and gratitude creates a solid foundation for inner peace and emotional balance.

By integrating these phrases into everyday life, each of them acts as an essential step on the path to self-healing. "I'm sorry" opens space for the recognition of one's own limitations and the acceptance of responsibility for everything that manifests in our lives. "Please forgive me" softens the relationship with the past and allows the release of guilt and resentment. "I love you" involves all experiences, including painful ones, with compassion and understanding, transmuting dense energies into lightness. Finally, "I am grateful" expands the perception of present blessings, connecting us with abundance and favoring the creation of a more harmonious reality. This continuous cycle not only transforms the individual but also radiates positive effects in all areas of life.

Practicing Ho'oponopono with dedication and conscious intention is to allow these four phrases to act as instruments of constant renewal. They do not require specific times or complex rituals; they can be repeated silently in times of challenge, written as daily affirmations, or integrated into meditation practices. Over time, this sincere repetition dissolves emotional and mental blocks, bringing clarity, serenity, and a deep connection with the divine essence. This process of continuous healing allows love and peace to flow freely, transforming the perception of life and opening paths to a fuller and more meaningful existence.

The phrase "I'm sorry" represents the first step in the Ho'oponopono healing journey. It is a sincere expression of acknowledgment and acceptance of responsibility for everything that happens in our lives. This acknowledgment does not mean taking the blame, but rather understanding that the memories and beliefs accumulated in our subconscious influence the way we perceive and interact with the world. Saying "I'm sorry" is an act of humility and courage, as it involves looking within yourself and admitting that, consciously or unconsciously, we contribute to the challenges we face. This phrase opens the doors to self-awareness, allowing us to recognize the limitations that prevent us from moving forward. By embracing our faults and imperfections, we create space for the beginning of transformation.

Next, the phrase "Please forgive me" emerges as a request for liberation. It is not about begging forgiveness from someone external, but about seeking reconciliation with one's own inner divinity, with that part of us that is pure, loving, and connected with the whole. This request for forgiveness is a gesture of deep respect and acknowledgment that negative memories and limiting patterns need to be healed. By saying "Please forgive me," we acknowledge that we are not perfect, that we make mistakes, and that we often carry unnecessary pain. It is also an invitation to let go of the shackles of the past, releasing guilt, regrets, and resentments. This forgiveness extends to ourselves and others, opening space for compassion and emotional lightness. Thus, we release the stagnant energy that prevents us from evolving and walk with more freedom.

The third phrase, "I love you," is the ultimate expression of unconditional love. This statement has the power to transmute any dense energy, involving painful memories with light and compassion. By repeating "I love you," we are not only referring to another person, but also to the parts of ourselves that need healing. This love is directed at our pains, our failures, our negative memories, and even challenging situations. To love these aspects of our experience means to accept the totality of who we are, recognizing that every part of us, even those we deem undesirable, deserves to be embraced. Love is a transformative force, capable of dissolving internal barriers and creating space for growth. It connects us with the universal flow of harmony and balance, allowing inner peace to settle in.

Finally, the phrase "I am grateful" completes the healing cycle with the energy of gratitude. By expressing gratitude, we recognize the abundance and blessings present in our lives, even in the face of challenges. This attitude puts us in tune with the natural flow of the universe, allowing more positive experiences to manifest. Gratitude not only reinforces the recognition of lessons learned but also strengthens the connection with the inner divinity. When we are grateful, we do not resist the present, but we accept it fully, recognizing that each experience has a purpose. Gratitude softens the mind, expands the heart, and keeps us aligned with abundance and harmony. Thus, it closes the cycle initiated by recognition, forgiveness, and love, consolidating the process of healing and transformation.

These four phrases, when repeated with sincerity and intention, create a powerful synergy. Together, they form a continuous cycle of recognition, release, transmutation, and gratitude. The consistent practice of this mantra does not require specific times or elaborate rituals; it is enough to integrate it into everyday life. It can be repeated silently in times of stress, in thoughts, written in diaries, or used as a focus in meditative practices. Over time, this constant repetition acts directly on the subconscious, dissolving emotional and mental blocks. This process does not eliminate life's challenges, but it transforms the way we relate to them, making us more resilient, compassionate, and centered.

The simplicity of these phrases is precisely what makes them so powerful. They access the deepest layers of the mind and heart, promoting a cleansing that is not only mental but also energetic and spiritual. This inner work is directly reflected in the way we deal with the outside world. Previously conflicting relationships become more harmonious, difficult decisions are made with more clarity, and challenges are faced with more serenity. The continuous practice of Ho'oponopono invites us to live more consciously, taking responsibility for our own reality and recognizing the power we have to transform it.

Incorporating this mantra into everyday life broadens our perception of the interconnection between our thoughts, emotions, and actions. Situations previously seen as obstacles begin to be perceived as opportunities for growth and learning. This change in perspective positively influences not only our personal lives but also the way we relate to others. The inner harmony we develop extends to our relationships, promoting empathy, understanding, and collaboration. Gradually, we become agents of transformation, spreading love and balance not only in ourselves but also in the environment in which we live.

By practicing Ho'oponopono consistently, we realize that each word spoken with intention is a firm step towards healing and self-knowledge. This continuous flow of love, forgiveness, and gratitude reconnects us with our divine essence and with the harmonious flow of life. The purification process that begins with "I'm sorry" and ends with "I am grateful" not only frees us from limiting patterns but also guides us towards a lighter, more authentic, and fuller existence. Thus, we walk with more clarity, allowing inner wisdom to guide us in every choice, in every step.

In this constant movement of cleansing and renewal, we discover that true peace is not in external circumstances, but in the harmony cultivated internally. Ho'oponopono, through its simple and profound mantra, reminds us that we have within us everything we need to heal, grow, and transform our reality. And so, we move forward, guided by the force of love, the power of forgiveness, and the abundance of gratitude, allowing each word chanted to be a link between us and the peace we so desperately seek.

With the continuous practice of Ho'oponopono, one realizes that the true power of these four phrases lies in the simplicity with which they access deep layers of the mind and heart. Each sincere repetition acts as a seed of transformation, cultivating a state of presence and balance. This process does not eliminate life's challenges, but it changes the way we relate to them, making us more resilient and compassionate. The inner harmony achieved is reflected in our actions, creating a lighter reality that is aligned with our essence.

By integrating the healing mantra into every aspect of life, we develop a broader perception of the interconnection between our thoughts, emotions, and the world around us. Situations that once seemed insurmountable come to be seen as opportunities for learning and growth. This more loving and welcoming outlook opens space for more authentic relationships and more harmonious coexistence. Gradually, we become agents of transformation, spreading peace and love not only to ourselves but also to those who cross our path. In this way, Ho'oponopono is revealed as a continuous practice of liberation and reconciliation. Each word spoken with intention becomes a step towards healing and self-knowledge. Thus, we continue walking with more lightness and clarity, allowing the flow of love, forgiveness, and gratitude to guide our choices. And, in this constant movement of purification and renewal, we discover the true essence of inner peace and the infinite capacity we have to transform our reality.

# Chapter 5
# Manifesting Your Desires

The human mind has an extraordinary potential to transform reality, directly influencing our thoughts, emotions, and actions. In Ho'oponopono, this power is channeled through creative visualization, a practice that allows access to and reprogramming of the subconscious mind to eliminate limiting memories and beliefs. This technique acts as an effective means of clearing internal blockages and creating a mental environment conducive to the fulfillment of desires and goals. By focusing attention on clear mental images charged with emotion, a neurological response is triggered that strengthens the connection between intention and action, driving concrete changes in everyday life.

The effectiveness of creative visualization is based on how the brain processes real and imagined experiences in a similar way. When a scene is mentally constructed with a wealth of sensory details, the brain responds as if that experience were actually happening, stimulating the creation of new neural connections and positively influencing behaviors and feelings. In the context of Ho'oponopono, this practice becomes even more potent when associated with the four fundamental phrases ("I'm sorry. Please forgive me. I love you. I'm grateful."), which promote deep emotional cleansing. This mental reprogramming process allows you to replace negative patterns with constructive thoughts, favoring the achievement of personal goals and emotional well-being.

By incorporating creative visualization into Ho'oponopono, it is possible to access areas of the mind that store memories and beliefs that limit personal growth. Consistent practice of this technique not only strengthens self-confidence, but also expands the perception of possibilities, creating a solid foundation for meaningful changes. This alignment between mind and emotion contributes to a genuine inner transformation, opening space for emotional healing and the manifestation of a more balanced, abundant, and harmonious life.

The power of the human mind is vast and profoundly influential in constructing the reality we experience. Within Ho'oponopono, this potential is channeled consciously through creative visualization, a practice that allows access to and reprogramming of the subconscious, dissolving limiting memories and beliefs that impede the natural flow of life. By using the mind to form vivid and emotionally charged mental images, a field of energy favorable to the manifestation of desires and goals is created. This process not only favors the achievement of goals, but also promotes a true inner transformation, allowing emotional and mental healing to happen naturally and continuously.

The basis of creative visualization is the principle that the mind does not distinguish between what is real and what is imagined. When we visualize with rich detail and involve that image with authentic emotions, the brain reacts as if it were really happening. This neurological response activates new neural connections, reinforcing positive behavior patterns and eliminating old conditioning. In the context of Ho'oponopono, this technique becomes even more powerful when combined with the four fundamental phrases: "I'm sorry. Please forgive me. I love you. I'm grateful." These sacred words act as a catalyst for clearing internal blockages, enhancing the process of manifesting a more harmonious reality.

By integrating creative visualization into the practice of Ho'oponopono, it is possible to access the deepest layers of the mind, where limiting memories and beliefs are stored. This access allows not only to recognize these patterns, but also to transmute them through love, forgiveness, and gratitude. Constant practice strengthens self-confidence, expands the perception of possibilities, and creates a solid foundation for meaningful changes. Thus, the alignment between thought and emotion becomes a powerful instrument of transformation, promoting the manifestation of a more balanced, abundant, and fulfilling life.

To use visualization effectively, it is essential to follow some steps that deepen the connection with the desired intention. The first step is to clearly define the goal you want to manifest. Having a detailed and specific vision of what you want to achieve is fundamental, as the mind responds better to concrete and sensory images. Then, finding a quiet environment where you can relax and focus your attention helps to deepen the experience. Closing your eyes, breathing deeply and allowing the mind to calm down is the beginning of this process.

During visualization, it is important to imagine the desired situation with all possible details: colors, sounds, smells, textures and, above all, the emotions that would arise when experiencing that experience. Emotion is the fuel of visualization, as it gives life to mental creation and strengthens the link between intention and manifestation. While visualizing, repeating the four phrases of Ho'oponopono - "I'm sorry. Please forgive me. I love you. I'm grateful." - further enhances the practice, clearing memories that may be blocking the path to fulfillment.

Gratitude plays a fundamental role in this process. Thanking in advance as if the wish has already come true reinforces trust in the flow of life and opens space for abundance to manifest. This genuine feeling of gratitude raises the energy frequency and aligns the mind and heart with the achievement of goals.

In addition to visualizing the fulfillment of desires, it is possible to apply creative visualization to clear limiting memories and beliefs. Imagining these memories as dark clouds dissipating in the sky or as stones being carried away by the current of a river helps to release these blockages in a light and fluid way. Feeling the lightness and freedom that this image provides reinforces the purification process and creates space for new possibilities.

To achieve consistent results with creative visualization, it is essential to maintain a regular practice. Dedicating a few minutes daily to this inner connection strengthens the habit and deepens the experience. Patience is also essential, as the manifestation of desires follows the natural rhythm of life. Trusting the process and keeping faith in fulfillment are attitudes that sustain the path. In addition, maintaining focus during practice avoids distractions and reinforces the clarity of intention. Combining visualization with positive affirmations further strengthens the belief in the ability to transform reality.

Over time, the constant practice of creative visualization combined with Ho'oponopono begins to produce noticeable changes. Small internal transformations are reflected in new opportunities, meaningful encounters and unexpected solutions that arise fluidly. This continuous alignment between mind, emotion and action strengthens the connection with the present, allowing desires to be nurtured with patience and trust.

This practice is not limited to a simple mental exercise, but becomes a way of life. Every thought, emotion and action becomes guided by the awareness that external reality is a direct reflection of the inner world. Thus, cultivating positive thoughts and elevated emotions becomes a way of aligning oneself with the best possibilities for the manifestation of desires. This process does not require excessive effort, but a conscious surrender to the flow of life, where clarity of intention and trust in the outcome are essential pillars.

As this understanding deepens, manifesting desires ceases to be just the achievement of external goals and reveals itself as a journey of self-knowledge and evolution. Ho'oponopono, combined with creative visualization, not only helps in achieving goals, but promotes a profound transformation. This transformation frees the being from limitations and opens space for a lighter, more authentic life aligned with the true essence.

Thus, each clean thought, each sincere emotion and each clear intention become seeds of transformation. These seeds blossom into a reality aligned with the purest essence of being, allowing life to flow with more harmony, balance and fulfillment. Ho'oponopono, by uniting healing and manifestation, leads us to a state of full presence, where each step taken is guided by inner wisdom and the creative power of the mind and heart.

By deepening the practice of creative visualization combined with Ho'oponopono, it is essential to understand that each thought and emotion emitted reverberates in the universe as energy frequencies. This vibration attracts similar experiences, shaping reality according to the quality of these energies. Thus, cultivating positive thoughts and elevated emotions is not just a mental exercise, but a way of aligning yourself with the most favorable possibilities for the manifestation of your desires. This process does not depend on excessive physical effort, but on a conscious surrender to the natural flow of life, where clarity of intention and trust in the outcome become fundamental pillars.

As this practice is integrated into everyday life, the perception of the circumstances around begins to transform. Small internal changes are reflected in new opportunities, meaningful encounters and unexpected solutions that arise fluidly. This continuous alignment between mind, emotion and action strengthens the connection with the present, allowing desires to be nurtured with patience and persistence. Visualization, then, ceases to be an isolated act and becomes part of a daily experience, where every choice and thought is guided by the awareness that external reality is a reflection of the inner world.

With this understanding ingrained, the process of manifesting desires reveals itself as a journey of self-knowledge and evolution. Ho'oponopono, combined with creative visualization, not only helps in achieving goals, but also promotes a profound transformation, freeing the being from limitations and opening space for a lighter and fuller existence. Thus, each clean thought, each sincere emotion and each clear intention come together to build a reality aligned with the true essence, allowing life to flow with more harmony, balance and fulfillment.

# Chapter 6
# Anchoring in the Present

Being fully present is a transformative experience that allows us to access inner peace and mental clarity, even in the face of daily pressures. Connection with the now not only calms the restless mind, but also strengthens the perception of the reality around us, promoting a state of balance and harmony. Conscious breathing emerges as an essential tool in this process, functioning as a direct link between body and mind. By directing attention to the flow of breath, it is possible to dissolve accumulated tensions, reduce anxiety and create an inner space of serenity, where emotions and thoughts are observed without judgment. This simple but profound practice offers us the opportunity to interrupt the automatic flow of worries and cultivate an authentic and tranquil presence.

The act of breathing deeply and consciously activates natural relaxation mechanisms in the body, reducing the stress response and promoting a sense of security and well-being. This state of calm not only benefits physical health, but also expands the ability to deal with emotional challenges in a more balanced way. By integrating conscious breathing into everyday life, it becomes possible to slow down the mental pace, allowing thoughts and feelings to flow more lightly and naturally. This process leads us to a clearer perception of ourselves and our reactions, favoring more conscious choices aligned with our true desires.

Cultivating present moment awareness through breathing creates an inner space conducive to self-knowledge and self-compassion. By anchoring ourselves in the present moment, we learn to value each moment and recognize the depth of simple experiences. This state of mindfulness strengthens the connection with our essence, promoting emotional healing and inner balance. Incorporating this practice into Ho'oponopono enhances its transformative power, as it allows us to clear limiting memories with more depth and authenticity. Thus, conscious breathing becomes a portal to a fuller, more peaceful life connected to what truly matters.

Breathing is the subtle and constant bridge that unites body and mind, an invisible flow of vital energy that sustains not only physical life, but also emotional and mental balance. With each inhalation, we absorb prana, the life force that invigorates the body, while exhalation carries with it not only carbon dioxide, but also emotional residues and accumulated tensions. However, when we are faced with moments of stress or anxiety, our breathing becomes short and rapid, reflecting the inner chaos and intensifying physical and mental discomfort. The body stiffens, muscles contract and the mind fragments, creating a vicious cycle of disconnection from the present.

It is in this scenario that conscious breathing emerges as a simple but profoundly effective antidote. By redirecting attention to the act of breathing, we are invited to perceive the air that fills the lungs, the gentle expansion of the abdomen and the calm release during exhalation. This deliberate focus anchors us in the now, dissolving the fog of restless thoughts and providing a haven of calm. Each breathing cycle becomes a subtle reminder that peace is always accessible, just a pause to reconnect.

The benefits of this practice extend broadly. Conscious breathing activates the parasympathetic nervous system, responsible for promoting relaxation and neutralizing the "fight or flight" response that is so wearing on the body. Anxiety slowly dissolves, replaced by a sense of security and stability. In addition, the mind becomes clearer and more focused, allowing for sharper concentration on everyday tasks. This mental clarity opens space for more thoughtful decisions and more balanced emotional reactions, avoiding impulsive and disproportionate responses to challenges that arise.

More than momentary relief, the continuous practice of conscious breathing deepens self-awareness. By observing the rhythm of breathing, we also become more attentive to the thoughts that arise, the emotions that cross us and the tensions that silently settle in the body. This gradual self-knowledge allows us to recognize emotional and behavioral patterns, creating the opportunity to transform them. Thus, emotions such as anger, fear or sadness cease to be uncontrollable forces and become experiences understood and processed with more serenity.

In the physical realm, the positive impacts are equally notable. Deep, rhythmic breathing increases oxygenation of the body, nourishing cells and organs more efficiently. This enriched flow strengthens the immune system, regulates blood pressure and improves cardiovascular health. The body, when fully supplied with air, responds with vitality and balance, directly reflecting overall well-being. Thus, taking care of breathing is also taking care of health in its entirety.

By anchoring in the present moment through breathing, the perception of life is transformed. Small details previously unnoticed gain meaning, and everyday life reveals nuances of beauty and depth. Each breath becomes an opportunity to give thanks for life, while each exhalation invites detachment and lightness. This state of mindfulness connects us more genuinely with the world around us, awakening a sense of belonging and harmony with the natural flow of existence.

There are several ways to cultivate this respiratory awareness. Abdominal breathing, for example, is a simple technique that can be practiced at any time. By placing one hand on the abdomen and the other on the chest, we are invited to perceive how the air fills the lower part of the lungs, promoting deeper and more complete breathing. This natural movement not only relaxes the body, but also quiets the mind, creating a space of tranquility.

Another powerful technique is alternate nostril breathing, which balances the hemispheres of the brain and stabilizes internal energy. By inhaling through one nostril and exhaling through the other in a rhythmic manner, the body and mind come into sync, dissolving tension and bringing mental clarity. This alternating flow softens extreme emotions and promotes a sense of centering, making it especially helpful in times of emotional turmoil.

The 4-7-8 technique also offers a simple and effective approach. Inhaling deeply through the nose for four seconds, holding the breath for seven seconds, and exhaling slowly through the mouth for eight seconds creates a rhythm that slows the body and calms the mind. This breathing pattern, repeated for a few minutes, acts as a natural sedative, being particularly effective in reducing anxiety and facilitating sleep.

Integrating these practices into the Ho'oponopono philosophy further enhances their effects. Before starting the repetition of the four phrases ("I'm sorry. Please forgive me. I love you. I'm grateful."), dedicating a few minutes to conscious breathing helps to clear the mind and establish a deeper connection with the present moment. During practice, breathing deeply with each phrase allows the energy of these words to penetrate more intensely, promoting a more authentic emotional cleansing. Breathing, in this context, becomes a channel to release painful memories and repressed emotions more gently.

In times of stress, combining conscious breathing with Ho'oponopono offers immediate and profound relief. By pausing and breathing with intention, we can repeat the four phrases as a mantra, allowing each word to intertwine with the flow of breath. This conscious movement gradually dissolves negative emotions, transforming discomfort into acceptance and serenity. Thus, the healing process takes place in a more organic and accessible way.

Allowing yourself to breathe with full attention is, therefore, a silent invitation to healing and self-knowledge. Each breathing cycle carries the potential to renew the body and clear the mind, dissolving emotional blockages and opening space for new perceptions. By uniting conscious breathing with Ho'oponopono, a fertile ground is created to welcome and transform emotions with delicacy, making the path of healing lighter and deeper.

This daily commitment to conscious breathing and cleansing words strengthens resilience in the face of adversity. Little by little, automatic responses and impulsive reactions give way to more thoughtful and conscious choices. The mind finds peace, the body relaxes and the heart opens to new possibilities. There is no demand for perfection in this process, only a gentle willingness to return to the present moment whenever necessary.

Over time, breathing with mindfulness ceases to be an isolated practice and becomes a natural habit. Breathing becomes a constant anchor that sustains emotional balance and physical health. Each moment lived with presence becomes an opportunity for inner reconciliation and renewal. Thus, the journey of healing reveals itself as a continuous flow of acceptance, love and gratitude. At this gentle pace, the simplicity of the act of breathing leads us, with lightness, to a fuller life deeply connected with our essence.

Allowing yourself to breathe with full attention is to open a silent path to inner healing. Each conscious breath carries with it the vital energy that renews, while each exhalation releases accumulated tensions and memories that no longer serve. This continuous flow of air not only sustains the body, but also purifies the mind, dissolving emotional blockages and clearing thoughts. By uniting conscious breathing with Ho'oponopono, a safe space is created to welcome repressed feelings and transform them gently, making the healing process more natural and profound.

This commitment to the present, sustained by breathing and the cleansing words of Ho'oponopono, strengthens resilience in the face of daily challenges. Gradually, it is noticed that automatic and impulsive reactions give way to more balanced and conscious responses. The mind calms down, the body relaxes and the heart opens to new perspectives. This state of presence does not require perfection, but rather a gentle willingness to return to the now whenever the mind wanders, cultivating a more compassionate view of oneself and life.

Over time, breathing consciously becomes a natural habit, a silent anchor that sustains emotional balance and physical well-being. Each moment lived with presence becomes an opportunity for inner reconciliation and renewal. Thus, the path of healing reveals itself not as a distant destination, but as a continuous process of acceptance, love and gratitude, where the simplicity of the act of breathing gently leads us to a fuller, lighter and truly connected life with essence.

# Chapter 7
# Deepening the Connection

Meditation is a powerful gateway to inner silence, allowing the mind to quiet down and the connection with one's true essence to strengthen. In Ho'oponopono, this practice becomes a profound path of healing and liberation, where thoughts and emotions flow freely, without resistance. By dedicating time daily to meditation, an inner space of tranquility and clarity is created, essential for dissolving limiting memories and opening space for new perceptions. This state of stillness not only promotes emotional balance, but also facilitates contact with inner wisdom, leading to a deeper understanding of oneself and the world around.

Integrating meditation with Ho'oponopono significantly amplifies the power of personal transformation. In this process, the mind becomes receptive to the repetition of the four fundamental phrases, enhancing the cleansing of unconscious patterns and creating a continuous flow of healing. The silence cultivated in meditation allows repressed emotions to surface in a light and natural way, promoting acceptance and forgiveness. Thus, the practitioner experiences a gradual release from negative thoughts, opening space for feelings of love, gratitude, and compassion. This inner harmony is reflected in the way each experience is lived, bringing lightness and balance to everyday challenges.

Meditating regularly provides a state of constant presence, where the mind is no longer dominated by past worries or future anxieties. This alignment with the present moment strengthens the perception of one's own existence and intensifies the connection with divine energy. By deepening the meditative practice combined with Ho'oponopono, it is possible to access more subtle layers of the subconscious, promoting a more effective cleansing of limiting beliefs. This journey of self-knowledge leads to a genuine transformation, allowing one to live with more authenticity, serenity, and fullness.

The human mind can be compared to a vast ocean, where waves of thoughts, emotions, and sensations alternate incessantly. On the surface, the waters are always agitated, driven by worries, fears, and desires. However, as we dive deeper, we find a space of serenity and silence, where turbulence does not reach. Meditation is this conscious dive into the depths of being, an invitation to quiet the mind and access the calmness that resides beyond the daily agitation.

When starting the meditative practice, we are gently led to observe our thoughts and emotions without the need to react or judge. It is as if we were sitting on the shore of this mental ocean, just witnessing the flow of the waves without letting ourselves be dragged by them. This simple act of observation allows us to create inner space, gradually dissolving the mental whirlwind and opening the way to inner peace. In this state of presence, the mind begins to calm down, and the connection with inner wisdom is strengthened.

The benefits of this silent journey are profound and comprehensive. Meditation reduces the production of cortisol, the stress hormone, promoting natural and deep relaxation. With constant practice, anxiety gives way to a stable tranquility, and the mind becomes less reactive in the face of adversity. The ability to concentrate and focus expands, allowing daily tasks to be performed with more clarity and efficiency. This renewed focus not only improves performance, but also favors more conscious and balanced decisions.

In emotional terms, meditation acts as a balm. It softens impulsive reactions and teaches how to deal with intense emotions in a more serene way. Anger, fear, and sadness cease to be dominant forces and become understood as passing experiences, which can be welcomed and processed without resistance. This emotional balance translates into more harmonious relationships and a more compassionate stance towards life.

More profoundly, meditative practice elevates self-awareness. By observing thoughts and emotions without interference, we develop a clearer understanding of our own internal patterns. We begin to identify limiting beliefs, automatic behaviors, and conditioning that often prevent us from moving forward. This recognition is the first step to transformation, because by illuminating these hidden areas, we open space for more authentic choices aligned with our true essence.

Meditation also expands spiritual connection. By silencing the mind, we approach a more subtle dimension of existence, where we can perceive the presence of the divine in us and around us. This experience does not require dogmas or specific beliefs; it is a natural feeling of belonging to the universal flow of life. This connection offers us comfort, inspiration, and a sense of unity with the whole, nurturing a serene trust in the journey we are on.

When we unite meditation with the practice of Ho'oponopono, this experience intensifies. The silence cultivated in meditation creates the ideal environment for the conscious repetition of the four sacred phrases: "I'm sorry. Please forgive me. I love you. I'm grateful." In this state of stillness, the words are not just spoken, but felt deeply, penetrating more subtle layers of the subconscious. Painful memories and limiting beliefs gently emerge into consciousness, allowing them to be embraced and dissolved with love and compassion. This continuous process of cleansing promotes a genuine transformation, freeing the being from invisible burdens and opening space for new possibilities.

Several techniques can facilitate this integration. Meditation with the four phrases is one of them. When sitting in a quiet place, with the spine straight and eyes closed, simply breathe deeply and repeat each phrase with intention. Feeling the meaning behind each word creates a healing vibration that spreads through the body and mind. Another approach is meditation with visualization, where we can imagine a serene and welcoming place, surrounded by a soft light that gently cleanses negative memories. Repeating the Ho'oponopono phrases in this internal environment enhances the purification process and renews vital energy.

Guided meditation is also a powerful tool, especially for those who are just starting out. Guides with a calm and compassionate voice, accompanied by soft sounds of nature or relaxing music, lead the practitioner through inner paths of healing and reconciliation. These guided practices offer safety and support, making the inner dive more accessible and welcoming.

For those seeking simplicity, meditation with a focus on breathing is an excellent choice. Observing the flow of air in and out of the body, feeling the expansion of the abdomen with each inhalation and relaxation with each exhalation, is a powerful way to calm the mind and cultivate presence. By integrating this conscious breathing with the Ho'oponopono phrases, each inhalation brings love and each exhalation releases pain, in a continuous cycle of renewal.

For the meditative practice to be truly effective, some attitudes can be adopted. Choosing a quiet environment, where distractions are minimal, is essential. Adopting a comfortable posture, keeping the spine straight, facilitates the flow of energy. Starting with a few minutes and gradually increasing the time avoids frustration. It is important to be patient and compassionate with yourself, accepting that the mind may wander and that returning to focus is part of the process. And, above all, regularity is fundamental.

Meditating daily, even for a few minutes, creates deep and solid roots on the path of transformation.

By allowing yourself to dive deeply into the practice of meditation integrated with Ho'oponopono, you access a dimension of peace and clarity that transcends rational understanding. Each conscious breath and each repetition of the sacred phrases dissolves old wounds, opens space for new understandings, and strengthens the connection with the essence. This process does not happen abruptly, but through subtle changes that, little by little, redesign the internal and external reality.

Over time, the cultivated silence becomes a constant ally. Life, once seen as a battlefield, becomes understood as a flow of experiences that teach and transform. Challenges lose the weight of insurmountable obstacles and become seen as opportunities for growth. Compassion flourishes, both for oneself and for others, creating an internal environment of acceptance and lightness that is reflected in all areas of life.

On this path of self-discovery, each moment of meditation becomes a reunion with one's own essence. The deep integration between Ho'oponopono and meditation reveals that inner peace is not a final destination, but a continuous state of being. Allowing yourself to experience this journey with surrender and constancy leads to a fuller life, where love, forgiveness, and gratitude become silent guides. And so, with a serene heart and a balanced mind, the mental ocean calms down, allowing life to flow with lightness, clarity, and authenticity.

By allowing yourself to dive deeply into the practice of meditation integrated with Ho'oponopono, it becomes possible to access a dimension of peace and clarity that transcends rational understanding. This state of silent surrender creates a fertile space for inner wisdom to manifest, guiding the practitioner through paths of healing and reconciliation. With each conscious breath and each repetition of the sacred phrases, old wounds begin to dissolve, opening space for a broader and more loving perception of one's own existence. This continuous process of cleansing and renewal transforms not only thoughts, but also daily attitudes and choices.

Over time, constant practice reveals that true transformation does not occur abruptly, but rather through subtle internal changes that, little by little, shape a new reality. The cultivated silence becomes a powerful ally, allowing the natural flow of life to lead to balance and harmony. Thus, challenges once seen as obstacles become understood as opportunities for growth and learning. Compassion for oneself and others flourishes, creating an internal environment of acceptance and lightness that is reflected in all areas of life.

On this path of self-discovery, each moment of meditation becomes a reunion with one's own essence. The deep integration between Ho'oponopono and meditation reveals that inner peace is not a destination, but a continuous state of being. Allowing yourself to experience this journey with surrender and constancy leads to a fuller life, where love, forgiveness, and gratitude become silent guides. And so, with a serene heart and a balanced mind, the mental ocean calms down, allowing life to flow with lightness and authenticity.

# Chapter 8
# Harmony in Bonds

Relationships are fundamental to our personal and spiritual growth, as they directly reflect how we relate to ourselves. Each interaction, whether with family, friends, romantic partners, or co-workers, offers a valuable opportunity for self-knowledge and evolution. Harmony in interpersonal bonds arises when we recognize that our experiences are shaped by internal memories and beliefs, often unconscious, that influence our reactions and behaviors. Taking full responsibility for these experiences allows us to transform conflicts into learning, creating space for more genuine and balanced connections. This process leads us on a journey of deep healing, in which we are invited to release judgments and expectations, promoting more authentic and enriching relationships.

The understanding that challenges in relationships are reflections of unresolved internal aspects opens doors to true transformation. Each disagreement or discomfort with the other signals the need to look inward and identify emotional patterns that perpetuate disharmony. This conscious look favors forgiveness, both of oneself and of the other, and encourages the practice of compassion and empathy. By dissolving resentments and releasing attachments, it becomes possible to establish healthier bonds, where acceptance and mutual respect prevail. This internal change reverberates positively in all interactions, making relationships safe spaces for growth and connection.

Adopting an attitude of gratitude for the experiences lived with the people around us strengthens bonds and promotes a lighter and more loving coexistence. Recognizing the value of each relationship, regardless of the challenges, allows us to see each person as a teacher who contributes to our evolution. This recognition motivates us to cultivate unconditional love, respecting differences and celebrating affinities. By transforming our perspective on relationships, we create an environment conducive to harmony, where understanding, open dialogue, and mutual respect are the foundations for lasting and meaningful relationships.

Each person who crosses our path carries with them a subtle reflection of who we are. Our relationships function as mirrors, revealing often hidden internal aspects, be they virtues or shadows that we need to embrace and transform. Whether in the family environment, in friendships, in love bonds, or in professional relationships, each interaction represents a valuable opportunity for learning and growth. When conflicts or discomforts arise, it is common to project the cause of these challenges onto the other. However, Ho'oponopono invites us to look inward and recognize that the roots of these conflicts often lie in unconscious memories and beliefs that we carry.

This ancestral practice guides us to take full responsibility for our experiences. Instead of seeking blame or justifying resentment, we are invited to reflect on which internal patterns are fueling disharmony. The conscious repetition of the phrases "I'm sorry. Please forgive me. I love you. I'm grateful" is not a simple ritual, but a profound process of healing. Each word carries with it the strength to cleanse the memories that generate expectations, attachments, and judgments. This internal movement releases the weight of the past and opens space for lighter and more authentic relationships.

Healing interpersonal bonds through Ho'oponopono does not mean ignoring limits or accepting harmful behaviors, but rather understanding that difficulties in relationships are opportunities for self-knowledge. When we take responsibility for our emotions and reactions, we become able to transform hurt into compassion and replace resentment with acceptance. This process does not require the other to change; the change begins within us and, consequently, reverberates positively in our connections.

Simple practices can strengthen this healing approach. Conscious communication is one of them. By practicing active listening, we seek to understand the other without judgment, paying genuine attention to their words and feelings. Expressing our needs with clarity and respect, without resorting to accusations, also contributes to a more harmonious dialogue. Nonviolent communication teaches us that it is possible to assert our limits and desires without disrespecting the other's space, creating an environment of mutual understanding.

Empathy and compassion are equally essential. Putting yourself in the other's shoes, trying to understand their pain and motivations, softens conflicts and brings hearts closer. Recognizing that we all face internal battles helps us to look at the other with more kindness. Forgiving, both ourselves and others, is another fundamental step. Forgiveness does not imply forgetting or justifying mistakes, but freeing oneself from the emotional weight that prevents evolution. When we choose to forgive, we open space for healing and renewal of bonds.

Another important aspect is the cleansing of expectations. We often expect the other to behave in a certain way or meet our emotional needs. However, each individual has their own path, and the freedom to be who they are must be respected. Releasing these expectations allows us to live lighter and more authentic relationships, where love is not conditioned by behaviors or results.

Cultivating gratitude also transforms the way we relate. Giving thanks for the people who are part of our lives, recognizing their qualities and contributions, strengthens bonds and opens the heart. Even challenges can be seen as gifts in disguise, as they teach us and make us grow. This grateful outlook makes relationships more harmonious and encourages us to value the presence of the other.

Visualizing harmonious relationships is another powerful practice. By mentally imagining positive interactions with the people around us, we are energetically building bridges of understanding and affection. Visualizing respectful dialogues, moments of joy, and gestures of affection contributes to the creation of a healthier emotional environment.

Ho'oponopono adapts to all types of relationships. In love bonds, the practice helps to heal emotional wounds, strengthen intimacy, and cultivate unconditional love. By taking responsibility for one's own emotions and expectations, it becomes possible to build a more solid and respectful relationship. Clear communication and mutual respect become essential pillars for the growth of the couple.

In family relationships, Ho'oponopono acts in reconciliation and healing of repetitive patterns that cross generations. Often, we carry ancestral memories that influence our behaviors and emotions. Practicing forgiveness and gratitude with family members, honoring ancestors and respecting differences, promotes unity and strengthens bonds.

Among friends, the practice encourages respect, trust, and reciprocity. Recognizing the qualities of friends, forgiving small flaws, and being a constant support makes friendships deeper and more meaningful. Lightness and joy flow naturally when there is mutual understanding and acceptance.

In the professional environment, Ho'oponopono contributes to a climate of respect and cooperation. The practice helps to dissolve conflicts and promote clarity in communication. Taking responsibility for one's own attitudes and maintaining an ethical and collaborative posture favors a more productive and harmonious work environment. Respect for differences and empathy with co-workers create a solid foundation for healthy professional relationships.

Building bridges in relationships requires courage and willingness to look inward. It is a continuous process of self-knowledge, forgiveness, and gratitude. By applying Ho'oponopono in our relationships, we transform not only the way we connect with others, but also the way we relate to ourselves. Each interaction becomes an opportunity for evolution, and each challenge, an invitation to grow with more love and awareness.

On this path of transformation, we realize that harmony does not mean the absence of conflicts, but the ability to face them with maturity and compassion. True harmony arises when we learn to respect differences, forgive imperfections, and value qualities. This internal balance is reflected in external relationships, creating more authentic and lasting bonds.

Thus, by committing ourselves to the practice of Ho'oponopono, we open space for lighter and more truthful relationships. Each "I'm sorry" is a step of humility, each "Forgive me" is a gesture of reconciliation, each "I love you" is a silent embrace, and each "I'm grateful" is a celebration of life. These simple but powerful acts of healing lead us to a more harmonious coexistence, where love and respect are the foundations that sustain our bonds.

Building bridges in relationships means cultivating connections based on mutual understanding, respect, and acceptance of differences. This construction requires a willingness to truly listen, communicate authentically, and keep the heart open, even in the face of challenges. Ho'oponopono helps us in this process by encouraging personal responsibility for our emotions and reactions, allowing us to dissolve emotional barriers and open paths for sincere dialogue. When we recognize that each interaction carries a purpose of learning, we begin to value bonds as opportunities for growth and joint evolution.

By consciously applying Ho'oponopono in relationships, we realize that we are not isolated in our experiences; we are part of a network of connections where every gesture, word, and thought has an impact. This perception inspires us to act with more kindness and empathy, understanding that harmony in bonds depends on the internal balance we cultivate. Thus, small acts of love, forgiveness, and gratitude transform the quality of relationships, making them lighter and more welcoming. With this, we begin to contribute to more peaceful and collaborative environments, both personally and professionally.

This journey of healing and reconciliation in relationships is not linear, but it is deeply enriching. The continuous practice of Ho'oponopono invites us to look at each bond with compassion and humility, recognizing that we are all in constant evolution. By committing ourselves to this process, we build solid bridges that sustain true and meaningful relationships. Thus, we learn that harmony in bonds begins within us and naturally expands to the world around us, nurturing connections that reflect love, respect, and authenticity.

# Chapter 9
# Healing the Roots

The family represents the foundation of our existence, being the first environment where we develop our perceptions about love, belonging, and coexistence. It is in this nucleus that we absorb behaviors, beliefs, and emotional patterns that shape our personal journey and directly impact how we relate to the world. Each experience lived within the family contributes to the construction of our identity and profoundly influences our choices and attitudes. Understanding that these family ties carry not only affections but also memories and traumas allows us to initiate a genuine healing process, where individual transformation reverberates throughout the entire family system, promoting harmony and balance.

By recognizing the depth of family connections, it becomes possible to understand that many challenges we face have roots in past stories and experiences, transmitted from generation to generation. We inherit not only physical characteristics but also emotional patterns and limiting beliefs that influence our decisions and relationships. Healing these patterns requires a compassionate look at the past, accepting that all family members acted according to their own limitations and circumstances. This understanding paves the way for the release of repetitive cycles and the construction of healthier relationships based on mutual respect, acceptance, and unconditional love.

When we propose to transform our relationship with the family, we take a significant step towards self-knowledge and personal evolution. The practice of forgiving, understanding, and welcoming differences allows us to dissolve hurt and resentment that often distance family ties. This conscious posture creates an environment conducive to open dialogue, strengthening emotional connections, and building a solid foundation of mutual support. Thus, by caring for these roots with love and dedication, we cultivate a family environment where understanding, empathy, and unity flourish, promoting a legacy of harmony for future generations.

The family is like a tree with deep roots, whose branches extend for generations, supporting and nurturing each new bud that blooms. From birth, we are immersed in this environment where we learn about love, belonging, and coexistence. The first impressions about the world, emotional bonds, and behavior patterns are shaped in this family space, profoundly influencing how we perceive ourselves and relate to others. However, just as a tree carries in its roots both strength and the marks of time, our family relationships also hold stories, beliefs, and emotional wounds that cross generations. Understanding this inheritance is the first step to healing the roots and transforming the present.

Ho'oponopono invites us to look at our family history with compassionate eyes, recognizing that all members of our lineage have carried, at some point, their own pains and limitations. Often, we inherit not only physical characteristics but also emotional patterns and limiting beliefs that influence our choices and shape our behaviors. Recurring conflicts, communication difficulties, and accumulated resentments can be reflections of old memories transmitted unconsciously. By bringing these patterns to consciousness, we open the possibility of interrupting repetitive cycles and initiating a healing process that benefits not only ourselves but our entire family tree.

Practicing Ho'oponopono in this family context is a profound gesture of love and responsibility. By repeating the four sacred phrases - "I'm sorry. Please forgive me. I love you. I'm grateful" - directed at family members or memories that generate disharmony, we initiate a process of energetic and emotional cleansing. Each sentence carries a powerful intention: to recognize our own limitations ("I'm sorry"), to ask forgiveness for thoughts and behaviors that contributed to conflicts ("Please forgive me"), to radiate unconditional love ("I love you"), and to express gratitude for the opportunity to learn and grow ("I'm grateful"). This internal, silent, and continuous movement begins to dissolve the invisible barriers that prevent reconciliation and understanding.

One of the first steps to healing these bonds is to develop conscious communication. This means listening actively, without interrupting or judging, seeking to understand the other's point of view with empathy. Expressing feelings clearly and respectfully, without accusations or demands, creates an environment conducive to open dialogue. Genuine listening allows the other person to feel valued and understood, while careful speaking avoids misunderstandings and resentment.

Forgiveness is another fundamental pillar on this path of healing. Often, we accumulate hurts that, over time, turn into emotional barriers, hindering the natural flow of love and coexistence. Forgiveness does not mean justifying harmful behaviors or forgetting what happened, but freeing oneself from the weight of the past. It is understanding that we all act, at different times, according to our own pains and limitations. By choosing to forgive, we give ourselves the chance to move forward with more lightness and openness to rebuild family ties.

Understanding and accepting differences is also essential to cultivate more harmonious relationships. Each family member is unique, with their own history, values, and ways of expressing feelings. Respecting this individuality, without trying to change or control the other, strengthens the foundation of the relationship. When we accept that everyone is at their own pace of evolution, we can deal with differences in a more compassionate and loving way.

To further deepen this healing process, the practice of visualization can be a powerful tool. Mentally imagining the family gathered in harmony, sharing moments of joy and connection, helps to create an atmosphere of peace and well-being. This visualization, accompanied by the Ho'oponopono phrases, enhances the cleansing of memories and contributes to building a more loving family environment.

Honoring our ancestors is also part of this healing journey. Often, we carry patterns and behaviors that are rooted in previous generations. By recognizing the influence of our ancestors on our history, we can express gratitude for all that we have received, but also choose to release patterns that no longer serve us. Ho'oponopono offers us the opportunity to send love and gratitude to past generations, promoting the healing of wounds that have been passed down. This gesture not only honors the legacy that has been left to us, but also paves the way for new generations to grow free from these conditioning.

The constant practice of Ho'oponopono within the family environment contributes to strengthening emotional bonds, promoting unity and understanding. As we cleanse painful memories and release resentments, we create space for unconditional love to flourish. This healing process does not require haste or perfection, but rather constancy and sincere intention. Each small internal change reverberates in relationships, transforming family dynamics gradually and significantly.

By caring for these roots with dedication, we cultivate an environment where empathy, respect, and love are nurtured daily. Small gestures, such as listening attentively, sincerely apologizing, or showing gratitude, are seeds that, over time, blossom into more authentic and profound connections. Thus, we transform the family into a safe space for mutual support and personal growth.

This journey of family healing is not limited to the present; it extends to the future. Each step taken towards understanding and forgiveness contributes to building a legacy of love and harmony that will be felt by those who come after us. The next generations will reap the fruits of this dedication, growing up in a lighter and healthier environment, where love and respect are fundamental values.

By committing to this transformation, we become guardians of a lighter and more loving emotional inheritance. Ho'oponopono reminds us that every conscious choice and every word of love has the power to transcend time, healing the past and illuminating the future. In this way, we honor our roots and allow our family tree to flourish with more strength and beauty.

Healing the roots is not erasing what has been lived, but understanding and transforming. It is recognizing that our stories, however challenging they may be, are part of who we are. And by choosing compassion and forgiveness, we offer ourselves and those we love the opportunity to rewrite this story with more love, balance, and harmony. Thus, we perpetuate a cycle of care and growth that will resonate for many generations, establishing a legacy of peace and unity.

By dedicating ourselves to this process of healing and reconciliation, we plant seeds of love that will blossom in future generations. Each gesture of understanding, each word of forgiveness, and each act of gratitude transforms not only our family experience, but also the path of those who will come after us. Thus, the cycle of pain and conflict gives way to a legacy of love, respect, and genuine connection, where each family member can grow freely, supported by roots strengthened by empathy and mutual care.

This movement of healing does not require perfection, but rather presence and true intention. Recognizing our limitations and those of others allows us to move forward with lightness, aware that each step taken in the direction of understanding already represents a great transformation. Over time, family ties are renewed, allowing new stories to be written, marked by trust, acceptance, and unconditional support. In this way, the family becomes not only a reflection of the past, but a safe space where love can manifest itself fully and authentically.

By embracing this path of healing, we become guardians of a lighter and more loving emotional inheritance. Ho'oponopono guides us on this journey, reminding us that every conscious choice and every word of love reverberates beyond us, reaching those who came before and those who are yet to come. Thus, we honor our roots and flourish as individuals and as a family, perpetuating a cycle of harmony and growth that will echo for generations.

# Chapter 10
# Freeing Yourself from the Chains

The past exerts a profound influence on our lives, leaving marks that can both strengthen and limit our growth. Painful experiences, traumas, and regrets accumulate like invisible chains that restrict our ability to live fully. However, it is possible to break these bonds and reclaim inner freedom through practices that promote reconciliation and emotional healing. Ho'oponopono emerges as a powerful path for this process, allowing us to transform difficult memories into learning experiences and free the heart from unnecessary burdens. This approach invites us to recognize and embrace each experience as an essential part of our journey, enabling a lighter and more harmonious life.

By integrating Ho'oponopono into everyday life, we develop the ability to take responsibility for everything that affects us, understanding that, even unconsciously, we participate in creating the circumstances we experience. This understanding does not imply blame, but offers the key to transforming our relationship with the past. Forgiveness becomes an indispensable tool, releasing resentment and allowing emotions like anger, fear, and sadness to be dissolved.

Through sincere acceptance, it is possible to realize that each experience, however challenging it may have been, has contributed to personal growth. This awareness opens space for gratitude, which softens the weight of memories and illuminates the path to new possibilities.

The constant practice of the four phrases of Ho'oponopono - "I'm sorry. Please forgive me. I love you. I'm grateful" - acts as an instrument of deep cleansing, facilitating the transmutation of limiting memories into positive energy. This conscious repetition envelops past experiences with love and understanding, undoing the emotional blocks that impede the natural flow of life. Thus, by releasing the shackles of the past, we open a space of peace and clarity that drives the creation of a future aligned with our true desires. From this state of balance, it is possible to build a new reality, guided by lightness, trust, and harmony.

The past, with its memories and experiences, often becomes an invisible burden that we carry throughout life. Unresolved traumas, regrets, and hurts create silent chains that bind us to limiting emotional patterns, hindering our ability to move forward and live fully. These emotional weights manifest as blocks, influencing our thoughts, behaviors, and decisions, preventing us from accessing our true potential. However, it is possible to break these bonds and reclaim inner freedom through emotional healing practices, such as Ho'oponopono, which guides us in the process of reconciliation with the past and the transformation of our most painful memories into learning and growth.

Ho'oponopono invites us to see the past with compassion, accepting that all experiences - good or bad - have played an important role in shaping who we are today. It is not about denying or forgetting what happened, but about embracing these experiences with love and understanding. The practice begins with personal responsibility, recognizing that, in some way, we participated in creating the circumstances we face, even unconsciously. This understanding does not bring guilt, but offers the power to change how we react to and relate to the past.

Taking responsibility is recognizing that we have the power to choose how we deal with our experiences. This means accepting that the emotions of anger, guilt, fear, and resentment that we carry are internal reflections that can be transformed. When we open ourselves to this understanding, forgiveness becomes a natural path. To forgive is not to justify what happened or erase the past, but to free ourselves from the weight that these negative feelings impose. It is an act of self-love that allows us to move forward with lightness and wisdom.

The conscious repetition of the four phrases of Ho'oponopono - "I'm sorry. Please forgive me. I love you. I'm grateful" - is a powerful tool in this process. Each phrase carries a specific intention that, when combined, acts in the deep cleansing of painful memories. When we say "I'm sorry", we acknowledge the pain we have caused ourselves or others. By asking "Please forgive me", we take responsibility for these pains and seek reconciliation. The statement "I love you" radiates unconditional love to ourselves and everyone involved, dissolving emotional blocks. And "I'm grateful" closes the cycle with gratitude for the lessons learned, allowing energy to flow freely.

This healing process can be enhanced through visualization. Mentally revisiting difficult situations from the past and surrounding the people and events with light and love contributes to the dissolution of emotional wounds. By imagining ourselves sending forgiveness and compassion to ourselves and others, we begin to fill the spaces previously occupied by hurt with serenity and understanding. This constant practice transforms how we relate to our memories, allowing us to move forward without the emotional weight that once limited us.

Accepting the past as part of our history is essential for healing. Acceptance does not mean resignation, but recognition that everything happened the way it needed to happen to bring us to this moment. This understanding opens space for gratitude, because even the most challenging experiences carry valuable lessons. Gratitude transforms the perspective on the past, softening the pain and bringing a sense of inner peace. When we are grateful for the experiences we have lived, we open space for new opportunities and paths previously blocked by the weight of memories.

By freeing ourselves from these emotional chains, we begin to perceive life more clearly. Decisions become more conscious and aligned with our values, and relationships are built from a place of authenticity and love. What once seemed like an insurmountable obstacle becomes a learning experience, and the past ceases to be a burden and becomes a silent teacher, whose lessons lead us to personal growth.

This healing process does not happen immediately, but develops gradually as we allow ourselves to experience each stage with patience and truth. Diving deep into oneself requires courage, but it also offers the opportunity to reconnect with our essence. Each time we choose to forgive, to give thanks, or simply to embrace a memory with compassion, we strengthen this connection and come closer to a more authentic and lighter version of ourselves.

With a lighter heart, we are able to see new possibilities. Paths previously obscured by fear or guilt are revealed, and life begins to flow more naturally. Decisions are made with more clarity, without the weight of old patterns. Relationships become healthier and more balanced, free from unrealistic expectations and conditioning from the past. And in this state of harmony, true freedom arises: the ability to create new experiences and live fully in the present.

Reframing the past is an invitation to write a new chapter in our history. A chapter where we are no longer prisoners of old pain, but conscious protagonists of our choices. The continuous practice of Ho'oponopono helps us to walk this path with lightness and love. Each "I'm sorry" brings us closer to humility, each "Please forgive me" reconciles us with our humanity, each "I love you" expands our heart, and each "I'm grateful" strengthens our connection with life.

This new beginning does not erase what has been lived, but transforms the way we carry our history. From this transformation, true freedom is born - the freedom to be who we truly are, without the chains of the past limiting us. With the past reframed and the heart at peace, we can finally walk with confidence towards the future, guided by the lightness of those who have understood that each experience was essential for the blossoming of their true essence.

Thus, the journey of freeing ourselves from the chains of the past is not just a process of individual healing, but an opening to a fuller, more conscious, and authentic life. By releasing the emotional ties that bound us, we allow ourselves to live with more joy, love, and gratitude, writing a new story marked by balance, harmony, and freedom.

This process of liberation does not happen instantly, but develops gradually as we allow ourselves to experience each stage with patience and authenticity. The constant practice of Ho'oponopono invites us to dive deep into ourselves, recognizing our weaknesses without judgment. This inner dive reveals hidden layers of emotions that, once embraced, become bridges to self-healing. Thus, each step taken towards forgiveness and gratitude strengthens the connection with our essence, allowing us to move forward with more clarity and purpose.

With a lighter heart, we are able to perceive new possibilities and paths that were previously obscured by the weight of memories. Life begins to flow more naturally, and choices that once seemed difficult become simpler and more aligned with our values. This state of balance gives us the freedom to create new experiences without repeating old patterns, opening space for healthier relationships, genuine achievements, and a more harmonious coexistence with the world around us.

By reframing the past and cultivating inner peace, we begin a new chapter in our history. A chapter where we are conscious protagonists, guided by the wisdom acquired and the lightness of those who have freed themselves from emotional bonds. With each new choice, we reaffirm our commitment to a fuller and more authentic life, where the past is just a step on the ladder of evolution, and the present becomes the fertile ground for new dreams and possibilities to flourish.

# Chapter 11
# Self-Esteem

Self-esteem is the essential foundation for a balanced and fulfilling life, directly reflecting on how we relate to ourselves and the world around us. Recognizing our own value and trusting in our own abilities are fundamental pillars for establishing healthy boundaries, facing challenges, and pursuing personal achievements. This process of inner strengthening requires overcoming limiting beliefs and negative memories that often obscure the perception of our intrinsic worth. Ho'oponopono emerges as an effective practice to dissolve these internal blocks, promoting self-compassion, forgiveness, and self-love as paths to develop a solid and authentic self-esteem.

Building healthy self-esteem involves looking inward with honesty and kindness, accepting our own imperfections and recognizing the qualities that make us unique. Past experiences, however challenging they may have been, have shaped our path, but they do not define who we are. By taking responsibility for our thoughts and emotions, we become agents of our own transformation. This internal movement allows us to free ourselves from self-critical judgments and patterns of comparison, favoring a more loving and respectful relationship with ourselves. This genuine acceptance creates a safe space for personal growth and the blossoming of new possibilities.

The constant practice of Ho'oponopono acts as a tool for emotional healing, capable of clearing memories that fuel insecurities and feelings of inadequacy. Through the phrases "I'm sorry. Please forgive me. I love you. I'm grateful," a deep process of inner reconciliation begins, which softens emotional wounds and dissolves accumulated guilt. This self-care strengthens confidence and connection with one's own essence, allowing self-love to flourish authentically. With this strengthened foundation, it becomes possible to move forward with courage in building a full life, guided by self-confidence and recognition of one's own worth.

Self-esteem is deeply influenced by our experiences, relationships, and the messages we absorb from the environment around us. From childhood, every word of criticism or rejection, every unfair comparison or negative experience can leave silent marks, shaping the way we perceive ourselves. These experiences can fuel insecurities, instill doubts, and perpetuate a feeling of inferiority that accompanies us throughout life. Often, these feelings become invisible roots that sustain limiting beliefs and hinder the recognition of our true value. However, it is possible to rewrite this internal story.

Ho'oponopono, an ancient Hawaiian practice, emerges as an invitation to reconciliation with ourselves. It teaches us that the true source of self-esteem is not in external opinions or material achievements, but in the deep connection with the divinity that dwells within each of us. By practicing Ho'oponopono, we initiate a process of inner cleansing, dissolving memories and beliefs that obscure our perception of value. This emotional purification opens space for genuine self-acceptance, allowing self-love to flourish naturally and confidence in our abilities to strengthen.

This path of strengthening self-esteem passes, first, through responsibility. Recognizing that we are responsible for the thoughts and feelings we cultivate about ourselves is a fundamental step. It is not about carrying guilt, but about understanding that we have the power to choose how we see ourselves and how we deal with our imperfections. This awakening leads us to the awareness that we can transform limiting beliefs and create a new internal narrative, more compassionate and empowering.

Forgiveness, in this process, takes on a healing role. Forgiving yourself for past mistakes, for failures, and even for not having protected yourself from certain situations is liberating. This practice dissolves the weight of guilt and silences the inner voice that criticizes and judges. Forgiveness opens the doors to self-compassion, creating a safe space for self-love to settle in genuinely. Thus, it is possible to embrace our imperfections without resistance, understanding that they are part of the human experience.

Self-acceptance is the fertile ground where self-esteem is strengthened. Accepting oneself fully, with qualities and flaws, is an act of courage and authenticity. This acceptance does not mean settling, but recognizing that we are beings in constant evolution. By accepting ourselves as we are, we pave the way for true and lasting changes, free from external pressures and based on respect for our essence.

This self-respect also manifests itself in the cultivation of self-love. Treating yourself with affection, respect, and understanding is a daily act that transforms the way we position ourselves in the world. Self-love is reflected in the choices we make, the limits we set, and the way we allow ourselves to live authentically. It becomes the solid foundation upon which we build a full and meaningful life.

Gratitude completes this cycle of inner strengthening. Being grateful for our own qualities, talents, and achievements puts us in tune with the abundance of life. Gratitude not only recognizes what we already have but also makes us realize how deserving we are of love, happiness, and success. This feeling expands our vision and strengthens the connection with our unlimited potential.

One of the most transformative practices of Ho'oponopono is the clearing of memories through the four powerful phrases: "I'm sorry. Please forgive me. I love you. I'm grateful." By repeating these words with sincerity, we create a movement of inner healing. They act directly on the emotional roots that sustain beliefs of inadequacy, dissolving fears, insecurities, and blockages. This loving dialogue with yourself restores confidence and brings clarity about who we really are, free from the distortions created by painful experiences.

Positive affirmations complement this process of rebuilding self-esteem. Declaring phrases like "I love and accept myself completely", "I am capable of achieving my dreams" and "I am deserving of love and happiness" reprograms the subconscious, replacing limiting beliefs with empowering thoughts. This daily habit creates new mental connections that support a more loving and confident vision of yourself.

However, for this process to be profound and transformative, it is essential to revisit and heal the wounds of the past. Often, emotional traumas, harsh criticism, and rejections experienced throughout life remain as open scars. Ho'oponopono invites us to look at these pains with compassion and understanding. By forgiving the people involved and ourselves, we dissolve the ties that keep us attached to these memories. This act of healing does not erase what has been experienced, but it reframes the past, freeing us to move forward with lightness and confidence.

Recognizing and celebrating one's own achievements is another essential pillar in building self-esteem. Every step taken, every obstacle overcome, and every lesson learned deserves to be valued. This celebration does not have to be grandiose; it can be a simple internal acknowledgment that we are moving forward. This habit strengthens self-confidence and reinforces the belief that we are capable of achieving our goals.

More than that, true transformation happens when we connect deeply with our essence. There is in each of us a pure, perfect, and unlimited part, which remains intact, regardless of external circumstances. When we silence the ego and tune in to this inner wisdom, we understand our intrinsic worth. This connection allows us to live with more lightness, authenticity, and unconditional love for ourselves.

This reunion with our own essence strengthens us in the face of adversity. We come to understand that criticism and rejection are part of the process of evolution and that our worth does not depend on the acceptance of others. This understanding brings serenity and allows us to establish healthy boundaries, prioritizing what truly makes us feel good. Choices become more conscious and aligned with our values, removing the need to please or fit into patterns that do not reflect who we are.

With strengthened self-esteem, we face challenges with more courage and confidence. Opportunities are embraced without fear, merits are recognized without guilt, and paths of personal fulfillment are followed with determination. Self-love becomes a safe guide, leading us to an authentic and rewarding life.

By practicing self-compassion and respect for our journey daily, we allow self-love to flourish naturally. Building solid self-esteem is an ongoing process, but each small step brings us closer to a lighter, fuller existence that is consistent with our true essence. On this journey, we learn to celebrate achievements with gratitude, face challenges with resilience, and above all, live with the certainty that we are fully worthy of love, happiness, and fulfillment.

This deep connection with our own essence allows us to see beyond the imperfections and limitations imposed by the external world. By recognizing that we are part of something greater, we understand that every challenge faced is part of our process of evolution. This perception strengthens us, bringing serenity to deal with criticism and rejection, as we come to understand that our worth does not depend on the approval of others. Thus, self-esteem becomes a reflection of the respect and affection we cultivate for ourselves, sustaining a solid foundation for us to live more fully and truly.

With the strengthening of self-esteem, we begin to position ourselves with more firmness in the face of life, establishing healthy boundaries and prioritizing what really makes us feel good. Choices become more conscious and aligned with our values, removing the need to please or fit into patterns that do not reflect who we are. This new perspective on oneself allows us to embrace opportunities with courage, recognize merits without guilt, and follow paths of personal fulfillment with confidence. Self-love is then revealed as an essential guide to building an authentic and rewarding journey.

By cultivating self-compassion and respect for our history daily, we give space for self-love to flourish naturally. The journey to true self-esteem is continuous and requires dedication, but each step on this path brings us closer to a lighter, fuller life aligned with who we truly are. From this solid foundation, we are able to face challenges with resilience, celebrate achievements with gratitude, and above all, live with the certainty that we are worthy of love, happiness, and fulfillment.

# Chapter 12
# Abundant Prosperity

True prosperity is revealed when we recognize that abundance goes far beyond material possessions, encompassing emotional balance, health, harmonious relationships, personal fulfillment, and inner peace. This state of fullness arises naturally when we are aligned with our essence and in harmony with the flow of the universe. The deep connection with our inner wisdom allows us to realize that we are deserving of a life rich in opportunities and happiness. By cultivating positive thoughts and nurturing feelings of gratitude, we attract favorable circumstances that drive growth in all areas of life.

Overcoming internal barriers is essential to allow prosperity to flow freely. Often, deep-rooted negative beliefs, such as the idea that wealth is inaccessible or that success requires extreme sacrifices, limit our ability to experience abundance. Identifying and transforming these beliefs is a fundamental step in releasing blockages and creating space for new possibilities. When we take responsibility for our experiences and recognize the power we have to reframe thoughts and emotions, we begin to build a more prosperous reality. This shift in perspective paves the way for developing a more open and receptive mindset to the opportunities that arise.

Integrating daily practices that reinforce trust in the flow of life strengthens the connection with abundance. Acts of generosity, positive affirmations, and the visualization of achieved goals contribute to establishing a healthy relationship with the concept of prosperity. Each inspired action, guided by intuition and purpose, brings us closer to achieving our goals. When we surrender to the present with trust and gratitude, we become co-creators of a full and balanced life, where prosperity manifests naturally and continuously in all aspects of being.

Many of the barriers that prevent us from experiencing true prosperity are deeply rooted in inherited or constructed limiting beliefs throughout life. From childhood, we are exposed to ideas that shape our perception of money, success, and abundance. Phrases like "money is dirty", "wealth is for the few" or "you have to suffer to win" become unconscious truths that limit our ability to prosper. These beliefs, often passed down from generation to generation or reinforced by negative experiences, create internal blocks that impede the natural flow of abundance.

However, Ho'oponopono emerges as a powerful tool for healing and transformation, allowing us to access and clear these memories stored in the subconscious. The practice invites us to recognize that these limitations are not part of our essence, but are merely emotional records that can be dissolved. By repeating the phrases "I'm sorry. Please forgive me. I love you. I'm grateful," we begin a process of releasing these beliefs, opening space for new possibilities. This internal movement creates a fertile environment for prosperity to manifest fully in all areas of life.

The first step in attracting true abundance is to take responsibility for our financial reality and the beliefs we hold about prosperity. It is not about blame, but about recognizing that we have the power to transform thoughts and emotions that limit us. When we understand that we are co-creators of our experience, we pave the way to reframe old patterns and build a more positive and receptive mindset to prosperity. This inner change is fundamental to dissolve energy blocks and allow the flow of abundance to reach all areas of life.

Gratitude plays an essential role in this process. When we cultivate gratitude for all that we already have - for our achievements, for the small daily victories, and even for the challenges that teach us - we come into tune with the energy of abundance. Gratitude expands our perception, allowing us to recognize the opportunities that are already present and attract even more blessings. This genuine feeling creates a positive vibration that connects us to the natural flow of prosperity.

Another fundamental element is the practice of visualization. Imagining yourself living a prosperous and abundant life, feeling the joy and gratitude for each achievement, is a powerful way to align the subconscious with our goals. By visualizing scenarios of success and fulfillment, we send clear signals to the universe that we are ready to receive. This practice strengthens confidence in one's own abilities and brings us closer to the desired goals.

Positive affirmations complement this journey of transformation. Phrases like "I am prosperous and abundant in all areas of my life", "Money flows to me with ease and joy" and "I deserve a life full of blessings" have the power to reprogram limiting beliefs. The constant repetition of these affirmations reinforces a positive mentality, undoing patterns of scarcity and installing new beliefs that favor prosperity.

The clearing of memories, through Ho'oponopono, acts directly on the emotional roots of limiting beliefs. By directing the four phrases to memories of scarcity, fear, and self-sabotage, we release stagnant energy and create space for new experiences. This healing process allows abundance to flow naturally, free from internal blockages. It is like opening doors that were previously locked, allowing new opportunities to enter our lives.

Generosity is also part of the virtuous cycle of prosperity. Sharing what we have, whether through donations, support for others, or acts of kindness, reinforces the flow of abundance. When we give with an open heart, without expecting anything in return, we demonstrate trust in the flow of life. This sincere act creates a chain of reciprocity, where what we offer returns multiplied.

However, prosperity does not manifest only through thoughts and feelings. Inspired action is essential to make dreams come true. Following intuition, acting with confidence, and taking advantage of opportunities that arise are fundamental steps to transform desires into reality. The combination of clear intention with consistent actions creates a solid path to success. Prosperity thus becomes a direct reflection of the conscious choices we make daily.

True prosperity is revealed when we balance all areas of life. Taking care of physical and mental health is essential to have the energy and disposition to take advantage of the opportunities that arise. Eating well, exercising, and cultivating healthy habits are ways to honor the body, our main instrument of manifestation. Likewise, investing in healthy and harmonious relationships strengthens our emotional foundation, creating an environment of support and well-being.

In the professional field, seeking work aligned with our talents and life purpose contributes to a sense of fulfillment and prosperity. When we dedicate ourselves to activities that bring us satisfaction, success becomes a natural consequence. This alignment between purpose and work generates not only financial return, but also a deep sense of contribution and meaning.

Spirituality complements this balance. Being connected with our divine essence and with the universe gives us clarity and direction. Spirituality reminds us that we are part of something greater and that abundance is available to all who allow themselves to receive. This connection guides us with wisdom and strengthens us in the face of challenges, keeping us firm on the path of true prosperity.

Allowing yourself to flow with the natural rhythm of life is to understand that abundance is not a finite resource, but an energy in constant motion. When we open ourselves to this flow, we realize that giving and receiving are part of the same cycle. Small acts of generosity, sincere gratitude, and actions guided by the heart create an energy field favorable to growth and fulfillment. This inner harmony is reflected in the opportunities that arise, allowing success to manifest in a light and spontaneous way.

By integrating Ho'oponopono and other conscious practices into our routine, we create a solid foundation for prosperity to flourish. Every thought free of limitations and every action taken with intention strengthens our confidence in life. Thus, we learn to trust the processes, understanding that each challenge brings valuable lessons and that each achievement is the result of our alignment with purpose.

Prosperity then ceases to be a distant goal and becomes an integral part of our daily journey. Living in abundance is recognizing that we are already complete and that true wealth manifests from the inside out. By freeing ourselves from limiting beliefs and opening ourselves to the natural flow of life, we become co-creators of a reality full of meaning and achievements. With a clear mind and an open heart, we are guided by a wise intuition that leads us to paths of growth, balance, and fulfillment. Thus, true prosperity is revealed as a natural state of being, where each moment is an opportunity to expand, share, and celebrate abundance in all its forms.

Allowing yourself to experience prosperity in its entirety is to understand that it is born from the balance between giving and receiving. When we open ourselves to this natural flow, we understand that abundance is not a limited resource, but an energy in constant motion. Small gestures of generosity, sincere gratitude, and actions guided by the heart create a positive cycle that expands the possibilities for growth. This state of harmony connects us with opportunities that previously went unnoticed, allowing success to flow lightly and spontaneously.

By integrating practices such as Ho'oponopono into our routine, we cultivate fertile ground for the flourishing of true abundance. Every thought free of limitations and every action taken with conscious intention strengthens confidence in our ability to prosper. Thus, we learn to trust in the processes of life, knowing that each challenge brings with it valuable lessons and that each achievement is a reflection of our alignment with purpose. Prosperity then ceases to be a distant destination and becomes part of our daily journey.

Living in prosperity is recognizing that we are already complete and that abundance manifests from the inside out. When we free ourselves from limiting beliefs and open ourselves to the flow of life, we become co-creators of a reality rich in meaning and achievements. With a clear mind and an open heart, we are guided by a wise intuition that leads us to paths of growth and fulfillment. Thus, true prosperity is revealed as a natural state of being, where each moment is an opportunity to expand, share, and celebrate abundance in all its forms.

# Chapter 13
# Inner Harmony, Healthy Body

True health manifests when there is balance between body, mind, and spirit, directly reflecting inner harmony and a deep connection with our divine essence. Every thought, emotion, and belief shapes the functioning of the physical body, significantly influencing our well-being. When we maintain positive feelings and cultivate constructive thoughts, we strengthen our vital energy, creating favorable conditions for physical and emotional balance. The search for complete health requires a conscious alignment between our inner attitudes and the way we interact with the world, allowing the body to respond with vitality and resilience. This state of harmony does not depend only on the absence of disease, but on a healthy integration of our physical, mental, and emotional aspects.

This balance begins with the recognition that we are responsible for our own well-being. By realizing how negative thoughts, stress, and repressed emotions can directly affect physical health, it becomes essential to cultivate practices that favor emotional and mental cleansing. The release of limiting beliefs and painful memories opens space for an energetic renewal that has a positive impact on the body. Thus, by nourishing the mind with positive thoughts and establishing a constant connection with our essence, we strengthen the immune system, balance our emotions, and promote the natural regeneration of the body. This continuous process of self-care and personal responsibility creates a solid foundation for comprehensive and lasting health.

Taking care of the body with healthy habits, respecting personal limits, and valuing moments of rest are fundamental pillars to sustain this state of balance. Balanced nutrition, physical exercise, quality sleep, and moments of relaxation contribute to physical and mental strengthening. By integrating self-healing and self-knowledge practices, we develop resilience in the face of challenges, prevent imbalances, and cultivate vibrant health. This holistic approach leads us to a fuller life, where body, mind, and spirit coexist in perfect harmony, reflecting a healthy and fulfilling existence.

Body and mind form a deeply interconnected system, where every thought, emotion, and belief directly impacts physical health. Stress, anxiety, fear, and resentment are emotions that, when not processed, create energy imbalances, manifesting in discomfort, illness, and physical exhaustion. Often, these accumulated feelings reflect old emotional patterns or limiting beliefs that block the natural flow of well-being. Thus, understanding this connection is essential to cultivating holistic health.

Ho'oponopono emerges as a transformative practice in this healing process, as it invites us to look inward and identify the memories and beliefs that cause disharmony. By repeating the phrases "I'm sorry. Please forgive me. I love you. I'm grateful," we begin a journey of inner cleansing, dissolving the negative emotional records that feed physical and emotional imbalances. This simple but powerful practice allows vital energy to flow freely, promoting not only physical health but also emotional and mental balance. Inner harmony is therefore restored, directly reflecting in the vitality of the body.

Taking responsibility for one's own health is a fundamental step on this path. When we recognize that our thoughts and emotions directly influence the functioning of the body, we become more aware of how to nourish our mind and spirit. This responsibility does not mean guilt, but rather the power to choose how to deal with the experiences and emotions we experience. This awareness allows us to make decisions more aligned with self-care, favoring the natural regeneration of the body and emotional stability.

Within this healing process, the practice of memory cleansing with Ho'oponopono plays an essential role. Directing the four phrases to memories related to illnesses, physical traumas, or negative beliefs about health creates an environment conducive to healing. By releasing these dense energies, we allow our body to activate its natural capacity for regeneration. This internal movement not only relieves physical symptoms, but also dissolves emotional patterns that could trigger new imbalances.

Visualization is a complementary practice that enhances this healing process. Imagining yourself with full health and vitality, feeling every cell of your body being bathed in healing light, reinforces the connection between mind and body. Visualizing the body functioning in perfect harmony strengthens confidence in one's own ability to heal. This technique, combined with the repetition of Ho'oponopono phrases, acts directly on the subconscious, reprogramming limiting beliefs and promoting well-being.

Positive affirmations also play a fundamental role in building solid health. Phrases like "I am healthy and vibrant," "My body heals and regenerates itself every day," and "I have energy and willingness to live fully" help reprogram the subconscious. By repeating these affirmations sincerely, we cultivate a mindset that favors physical and emotional balance. This continuous process of inner strengthening is reflected in increased disposition, vitality, and physical endurance.

Gratitude for the body and for health is another essential pillar in this journey. When we recognize and give thanks for the functioning of our body, even in the face of challenges, we send a message of love and appreciation to every cell. Gratitude has the power to strengthen the immune system and create an internal environment conducive to healing. This sincere feeling of appreciation for our body connects us with the energy of abundance and well-being.

However, for this harmony to be maintained, it is necessary to adopt healthy lifestyle habits. A balanced diet, rich in nutrients, combined with regular physical exercise, quality sleep, and contact with nature, creates a solid foundation for the balance of body and mind. This physical care is complemented by emotional self-care, which includes moments of relaxation, meditation, and practices that provide pleasure and well-being. Self-care is an expression of self-love that nourishes all aspects of being.

Ho'oponopono can also be used as a complementary tool in the treatment of physical and emotional illnesses. By clearing memories and beliefs related to illnesses, we open space for healing to manifest on deep levels. Although it does not replace conventional medical treatments, this practice enhances healing processes by acting directly on the emotional and energetic causes of diseases. The integration between medical care and self-healing practices expands the possibilities for recovery and balance.

Mental health, as important as physical health, also benefits enormously from Ho'oponopono. Problems such as stress, anxiety, and depression often have roots in painful memories and distorted beliefs about ourselves. By clearing these memories, we cultivate inner peace, emotional balance, and serenity. This process strengthens resilience in the face of challenges, allowing us to deal with emotions in a healthier and more constructive way.

Seeking holistic health is, therefore, cultivating a state of harmony between body, mind, and spirit. This balance invites us to take care of all aspects of our being, nurturing the connection with our divine essence. True healing happens when we recognize this integration and begin to act in alignment with it. Thus, every positive thought, every emotion welcomed, and every gesture of self-care contributes to the construction of vibrant and sustainable health.

When we understand that healing begins within, each step towards self-knowledge and self-care takes on new meaning. Practices like Ho'oponopono not only relieve physical and emotional pain, but also guide us on a profound journey of reconciliation with ourselves. This constant cleansing allows vital energy to circulate freely, nourishing the body, balancing the mind, and uplifting the spirit. Every gesture of self-love, however small, becomes a powerful link in building holistic health.

Integrating these practices into daily routine means being attentive to the body's signals and the emotions that arise, welcoming them with compassion and understanding. Small changes, such as setting aside time to silence the mind, eating consciously, or practicing regular exercise, become big steps towards balance. From this perspective, health is no longer seen just as the absence of disease, but as a direct reflection of the harmony between our inner and outer worlds.

Walking this path of balance and self-healing awakens us to the understanding that we are co-creators of our own reality. This understanding inspires us to respect the body, nourish the mind with constructive thoughts, and nurture the spirit with love. Thus, we achieve a state of fullness where health flourishes naturally, guiding us to a lighter, more balanced life, deeply connected with who we truly are.

When we understand that true healing is born from within, we begin to value every step taken towards self-knowledge and self-care. Practices such as Ho'oponopono not only relieve emotional and physical pain, but also lead us on a profound journey of reconciliation with ourselves. This process of cleansing and renewal allows vital energy to flow freely, promoting not only the recovery of the body, but also the strengthening of the mind and spirit. Thus, every gesture of self-love is transformed into an essential link in building comprehensive and lasting health.

Integrating these practices into everyday life means being attentive to the body's signals and the emotions that emerge, welcoming them with compassion and understanding. Small changes, such as setting aside time to meditate, eating consciously, and cultivating positive thoughts, become powerful instruments of transformation. From this new perspective, health is no longer seen just as the absence of disease and becomes recognized as a direct reflection of the harmony between our inner and outer worlds.

By walking this path of balance and self-healing, we awaken to the awareness that we are co-creators of our own reality. This understanding inspires us to take care of the body with respect, nourish the mind with wisdom, and nurture the spirit with love. Thus, we achieve a state of fullness where health flourishes naturally, guiding us to a lighter, more balanced life, deeply connected with our essence.

# Chapter 14
# Inner Flow

Creativity is an energy inherent in all human beings, a natural flow that arises from a deep connection with one's own essence. It manifests itself in multiple ways, whether in art, music, science, problem solving, or the creation of innovative ideas. This creative force does not depend on exceptional talents, but on the ability to access and allow this energy to flow freely. When we align our thoughts and emotions with this inner force, we become capable of transforming ideas into reality, finding original solutions, and expressing our individuality in an authentic way.

In the creative development process, it is common for emotional and mental obstacles to arise, limiting the full expression of this potential. Negative beliefs, fears, and insecurities are barriers that restrict creative flow and distance the connection with genuine inspiration. By recognizing these blockages as accumulated memories and patterns, it is possible to initiate a process of cleansing and release, allowing creativity to manifest spontaneously and without limitations. Thus, the path opens to a freer, lighter expression, connected with the inner essence.

By cultivating a state of presence and openness, the mind becomes more receptive to new ideas and perspectives. This state favors intuition, which emerges as a natural guide for creation and innovation. From this authentic connection, creativity becomes a channel for expressing the true essence, driving actions that reflect balance, harmony, and purpose. Creative fluidity is not just a skill, but a natural expression of being, capable of transforming the way we relate to the world and ourselves.

Creativity is a natural and unlimited expression of the human essence, a vital energy that flows when we are in harmony with our inner self. It is not restricted to artistic skills or extraordinary talents, but manifests itself in countless ways in everyday life - be it in art, science, problem solving or the creation of new ideas. This creative force emerges spontaneously when we allow ourselves to access our inner wisdom and trust our intuition. However, many of us block this creative flow due to limiting beliefs, fears and insecurities, which function as invisible barriers, preventing the free manifestation of our creative potential.

Ho'oponopono offers a path to unblock this creative energy. This Hawaiian practice of reconciliation and emotional cleansing teaches that memories and beliefs stored in the subconscious can be cleansed, allowing creativity to flow unimpeded. The four phrases - "I'm sorry. Please forgive me. I love you. I'm grateful." - function as an internal purification process. By directing these words to memories of criticism, rejection, or fears related to creative expression, we dissolve internal resistance and open space for new ideas to emerge with lightness and authenticity. This ongoing practice not only removes blockages, but also strengthens the connection with intuition, a powerful source of inspiration.

Connecting with intuition is essential to accessing creative flow. Intuition, often silenced by excessive rationality or fear of making mistakes, is the voice of inner wisdom, capable of guiding our creations with clarity and purpose. To hear it, it is necessary to silence the mind, slow down and allow yourself to be present. This state of presence favors the perception of new ideas and perspectives, making the creative process more fluid and spontaneous. When we trust this inner voice, we are guided to paths of innovation and genuine expression.

Visualization is another powerful tool to stimulate creativity. By imagining yourself creating with freedom and joy, visualizing projects being completed or ideas being developed, we strengthen the link between mind and action. Visualizing the realization of artistic creations, innovative solutions or new possibilities reinforces confidence in our creative capacity. This practice sends clear signals to the subconscious that we are ready to transform ideas into reality, making the creative process more accessible and natural.

Positive affirmations complement this unblocking process. Phrases such as "I am creative and inspired", "Creativity flows freely through me" and "I express my ideas with confidence" act as commands that reprogram the subconscious. The constant repetition of these affirmations dissolves negative beliefs and strengthens the conviction that we are fully capable of creating. This positive inner dialogue builds a solid foundation for creativity to flourish without restriction.

In addition to mental and emotional practices, experimentation is fundamental to releasing creative flow. Allowing yourself to explore different techniques, materials and forms of expression is an invitation to the new and the unknown. This openness to experimentation reduces the fear of failure and encourages the discovery of new paths. Often, creativity arises precisely when we move away from the pursuit of perfection and surrender to the process with lightness and curiosity.

Nature is also an inexhaustible source of inspiration. Observing the harmony, diversity and simplicity of natural cycles awakens creative insights and renews the mind. Walks in the open air, contemplation of landscapes or simply listening to the sound of water and winds are ways to reconnect with the natural flow of life, bringing clarity and new ideas. Connection with nature calms the mind and opens space for creativity to manifest spontaneously.

Cultivating curiosity is equally essential to nurturing the creative process. Being open to new experiences, knowledge and perspectives expands the internal repertoire and stimulates the mind to seek unconventional solutions. Curiosity drives us to question, explore and reinvent, fundamental characteristics for innovation and creation. This curious look at the world around us invites us to see possibilities where we once saw limitations.

When we remove internal blocks and reconnect with intuition, creativity flows like a river free of obstacles. Ho'oponopono facilitates this cleansing process, creating a clean and receptive inner space for new ideas. This state of openness allows us not only to create, but also to transform the way we live and relate to the world. Creativity ceases to be an occasional skill and becomes a constant force for renewal and evolution.

Incorporating creativity into everyday life is a continuous exercise in self-knowledge and expression. From small daily decisions to large projects, creativity can be applied in various areas of life - at work, in relationships, in problem solving and in personal development. This integration makes living more authentic and meaningful, as each action begins to reflect our true essence.

When we surrender to the creative flow, we open ourselves to a journey of self-discovery. Each materialized idea, each completed creation is an extension of who we are, a reflection of our inner truth. This process not only expands our possibilities, but also invites us to reinvent paths and manifest our uniqueness in a genuine way. Creativity thus becomes a bridge between our inner world and external reality, allowing us to contribute significantly to the world around us.

By integrating practices such as Ho'oponopono, visualization and positive affirmations, we create an internal environment conducive to creative awakening. This environment strengthens us emotionally, allowing us to face challenges with lightness and confidence. The mind expands, new ideas emerge and innovative solutions arise naturally. This movement inspires us to explore unknown territories and transform challenges into opportunities, awakening an unlimited creative potential.

In this way, creativity is consolidated as a powerful link between our being and the world. It drives us to live with purpose, to create with intention and to express our truth authentically. By nurturing this inner flow, we not only bring our ideas to life, but also become agents of change. We are able to inspire others to also explore their creativity, creating a continuous cycle of innovation and transformation.

Thus, creativity is revealed not as a sporadic resource, but as a constant force that guides us towards a richer, more meaningful life, aligned with our essence. When we allow ourselves to flow with this creative energy, we open doors to infinite possibilities and to the realization of our most authentic dreams.

When we allow creativity to flow without barriers, we open the way to a journey of self-discovery and transformation. Each conceived idea and each authentic expression reflect not only our individuality, but also the connection with something greater, which transcends limits and patterns. This continuous flow of creation invites us to explore new possibilities, reinvent paths and manifest our essence in everything we do. Thus, creativity ceases to be a sporadic resource and becomes a constant force for renewal and evolution.

By integrating emotional cleansing practices, such as Ho'oponopono, and cultivating states of presence and curiosity, we learn to deal with creative challenges in a lighter and more confident way. The mind expands, opening space for innovative ideas and solutions that previously seemed unattainable. This process strengthens us internally and inspires us to explore new territories, awakening an unlimited creative potential that transforms our relationship with the world and with ourselves.

In this way, creativity is established as a bridge between our inner self and the reality around us. It drives us to live with purpose, to build with meaning and to express our truth in a genuine way. By nurturing this inner flow, we not only bring our ideas to life, but also become agents of change, capable of transforming challenges into opportunities and inspiring others to follow the same path of authentic expression and fulfillment.

# Chapter 15
# Legacies of the Past

Ancestry is deeply integrated into our existence, shaping who we are through the stories, traditions, and memories passed down by our ancestors. Every experience lived by previous generations is reflected in our behaviors, beliefs, and daily decisions, silently influencing the way we lead our lives. This invisible connection is not limited to positive legacies, but also involves dysfunctional patterns, unresolved pain, and limiting beliefs that continue to manifest over time. Recognizing and understanding this influence is essential to promote inner healing and unleash the potential to live with more lightness and authenticity. Ho'oponopono emerges as an effective way to access these inherited memories, allowing emotional and spiritual cleansing that reverberates throughout the family lineage.

By taking responsibility for these transmitted patterns, even those we do not fully understand, we create the opportunity to break repetitive cycles and transform our reality. The practice of Ho'oponopono, with its words of repentance, forgiveness, love, and gratitude, offers a compassionate approach to dealing with ancestry, recognizing that the choices and attitudes of our ancestors were shaped by the circumstances of their times. This process does not seek to judge or justify the past, but rather to embrace it with understanding and promote the necessary healing to move forward. Freeing ourselves from these limiting memories allows us to open space for a new perspective on life, more aligned with well-being, harmony, and personal growth.

By integrating this practice of forgiveness and reconciliation into our journey, we not only transform our own experience, but also positively impact our family and future generations. Ho'oponopono becomes a bridge between past, present, and future, encouraging us to honor the legacy received, while consciously choosing to build a healthier and more balanced path. This movement of ancestral healing strengthens our connection to our family roots and empowers us to create an environment where abundance, love, and peace can flourish genuinely and lastingly.

The experiences, beliefs, and emotions lived by our ancestors shape, in a subtle and profound way, how we lead our lives. Emotional and behavioral inheritances are transmitted through untold stories, repetitive family patterns, and unconscious behaviors that influence our choices. Many of these influences are invisible, as they are rooted in emotional memories that span generations, creating cycles of repetition of traumas, limiting beliefs, and difficulties that seem to perpetuate themselves. Understanding this ancestral connection is essential so that we can identify and transform the patterns that prevent us from living fully.

Ho'oponopono presents itself as an effective practice to access and cleanse these inherited memories. It invites us to take responsibility not only for our own thoughts and actions, but also for the family memories that we carry unconsciously. The practice of the four phrases - "I'm sorry. Please forgive me. I love you. I'm grateful." - acts as a balm on these ancestral wounds, promoting emotional and spiritual healing that reverberates throughout our lineage. This process does not seek to justify or erase the past, but to embrace it with compassion, understanding that our ancestors did the best they could within the circumstances of their time.

Forgiving the ancestral past is an act of profound liberation. It does not mean denying or minimizing the pain and challenges experienced by previous generations, but recognizing that, like us, they were also influenced by their own contexts and limitations. When we direct the words of Ho'oponopono to our ancestors, we acknowledge these pains and, at the same time, open space for healing. This gesture of love and understanding dissolves invisible bonds, allowing repetitive patterns to be interrupted and new possibilities to flourish in our lives.

By recognizing inherited patterns, such as financial difficulties, dysfunctional relationships, or self-limiting beliefs, we can begin the transformation process. Ho'oponopono invites us to observe these cycles with attention and direct the cleansing practice to these aspects. This release creates an internal space for more conscious choices aligned with our desires and purposes. Thus, we cease to be hostages to a repetitive history and become authors of our own narrative.

Honoring ancestral legacy is a fundamental part of this process. Recognizing the strength, resilience, and wisdom of our ancestors does not erase their flaws, but expands our understanding of who we are. We can cultivate this honor through the preservation of family traditions, the appreciation of the stories that have been told to us, and gratitude for the journey that has brought us this far. This recognition not only strengthens our identity, but also builds a solid foundation for us to move forward with more confidence and balance.

Healing the family tree is an act that transcends the individual. By cleansing memories and limiting patterns, we promote healing not only for ourselves, but for our entire lineage, also impacting future generations. Breaking negative cycles means offering our descendants a lighter and more harmonious legacy. This healing process is a gift that echoes through time, allowing love, wisdom, and prosperity to flow freely through the generations.

This journey of reconciliation with the ancestral past reinforces the awareness that we are living links in a chain that runs through time. Every act of healing and forgiveness we perform reverberates silently, positively impacting not only our lives, but also the lives of those who came before and those who are yet to come. By freeing ourselves from inherited pain, we allow our lineage to move towards a path of more love, balance, and abundance.

Integrating this practice into our daily lives is an exercise in presence and responsibility. Observing how certain recurring behaviors or emotions may be linked to family memories is the first step to healing. With each recognition, we can apply Ho'oponopono, bringing lightness and compassion to these experiences. This constant practice allows us to undo emotional knots and rebuild our paths more consciously.

This healing movement also brings us closer to a deeper understanding of the nature of compassion. When we look at the past with empathy, we realize that, like us, our ancestors faced challenges and made decisions based on their own limitations and contexts. This understanding frees us from the burden of judgment and invites us to walk a path of understanding and acceptance, both in relation to the past and the present.

By freeing ourselves from these emotional inheritances, we begin to build a more authentic and lighter life. The absence of repetitive patterns allows new choices to be made from a place of clarity and alignment with our essence. Thus, our relationships become healthier, our decisions more conscious, and our path more aligned with our true values.

This process also inspires us to create a positive legacy. By healing the wounds of the past, we leave a trail of love, wisdom, and freedom for those who will follow after us. Our descendants will inherit not only stories, but also the strength of a lineage that chose to break with patterns of pain and build a solid foundation of love and understanding. This is the true power of ancestral healing: to transform not only the present, but to shape a lighter and more prosperous future.

Allowing yourself to honor and heal the past is an act of courage and love. Choosing this path is recognizing that each step of healing strengthens our journey and enriches the world around us. Thus, the legacy we leave becomes marked by balance, compassion, and authenticity. We are invited to live more consciously, free from the burdens that no longer belong to us, and to offer the world our best version.

Thus, by integrating Ho'oponopono as a tool for ancestral healing, we access a state of deep balance and connection with our roots. This practice allows us to transform pain into wisdom, weight into lightness, and repetition into freedom. We are then able to build a life in harmony with our essence and leave a legacy of love and awareness for generations to come.

By freeing ourselves from inherited burdens and limiting memories, we create space for new possibilities to flourish in our lives and in the lives of our descendants. This healing process not only dissolves repetitive patterns, but also strengthens our identity and reconnects us with ancestral wisdom in a lighter and more conscious way. Thus, we become free to build a future guided by balance, abundance, and healthier relationships, where the past no longer dictates our path, but inspires choices more aligned with our true essence.

This journey of reconciliation with ancestry reminds us that we are living links in a chain that runs through time. Every act of forgiveness and love dedicated to our ancestors silently reverberates in all directions, touching past and future generations. By healing our history, we not only liberate ourselves, but also offer a purer and more harmonious legacy for those to come. This transformation is reflected in new ways of thinking, feeling, and acting, creating solid roots for the flourishing of a fuller existence.

Allowing yourself to heal and honor the past is a gesture of courage and love. By choosing this path, we are not only ending cycles of pain, but opening doors to more authentic and meaningful experiences. We are invited to live with more compassion and awareness, recognizing that each step of healing and liberation strengthens our journey and enriches the world around us. Thus, the legacy we leave becomes marked by love, wisdom, and freedom, guiding us to a truly renewed future.

# Chapter 16
# Ho'oponopono for Children

Ho'oponopono presents itself as an essential tool to support the emotional and spiritual development of children, providing them with resources to deal with feelings and challenges from an early age. By being introduced to this practice, they learn to recognize and understand their emotions, cultivating responsibility for their thoughts and attitudes. This approach favors the construction of a solid foundation for self-knowledge and empathy, allowing children to develop more harmonious relationships and deal positively with adverse situations. The simplicity and depth of Ho'oponopono make this philosophy accessible and transformative, awakening in children the ability to promote their own healing and positively impact the environment around them.

Integrating Ho'oponopono into children's routines stimulates the awareness that every action and thought has an impact on their lives and the world. The practice of the phrases "I'm sorry, please forgive me, I love you, I'm grateful" teaches fundamental values such as forgiveness, gratitude, and self-love, elements that strengthen self-esteem and encourage compassionate attitudes. By learning to take responsibility for their emotions and transform negative feelings, children develop skills to face conflicts with maturity and balance, building a healthy emotional foundation that will accompany them throughout their lives.

This learning process not only benefits individual growth, but also contributes to a more harmonious family and social environment. Children who practice Ho'oponopono become examples of empathy, respect, and cooperation, positively influencing those around them. Thus, the introduction of this practice in childhood not only favors the emotional well-being of children, but also promotes a culture of peace and understanding, forming more aware individuals who are prepared to build a better future.

Children, by nature, are receptive spirits, with hearts still free from many limiting conditions and beliefs. This inner purity makes them absorb new teachings with ease and naturalness. In this context, Ho'oponopono emerges as a particularly accessible practice for children, as its simplicity and depth can be presented in a playful and creative way. When led by engaging stories or activities that stimulate the imagination, children awaken to the awareness that they are powerful beings, fully capable of transforming themselves and the world around them. This discovery reinforces the idea that every thought, feeling, and action directly influences the reality they experience.

To make Ho'oponopono truly meaningful for children, it is essential to adapt the language and concepts to their understanding. The introduction of this philosophy should be done in a light and fun way, using resources that stimulate the natural interest of children. Enchanting stories, engaging games, colorful drawings, and captivating songs are effective tools to convey the principles of this practice. By exploring these resources, children can more easily assimilate the importance of taking responsibility for their thoughts and emotions, learning to identify and transform feelings of sadness, anger, or fear.

Simple language is fundamental in this process. Explaining the principles of Ho'oponopono clearly, with words that children understand, facilitates understanding. Talking about how thoughts and emotions influence their actions and how it is possible to "cleanse" memories that cause discomfort creates a safe space for reflection. For example, describing painful memories as "little monsters" that live hidden in the mind makes it easier for the child to understand that these feelings can be embraced with love and gratitude, transforming them into "friends" that no longer cause pain.

Stories and metaphors play a crucial role in this learning. Narratives that feature characters facing emotional challenges and overcoming them with the practice of Ho'oponopono help children visualize how this tool can be applied in their own lives. An example would be to tell the story of a character who feels afraid to sleep alone, but learns to talk to his thoughts and emotions through the phrases "I'm sorry, please forgive me, I love you, I'm grateful", transforming fear into courage and tranquility. These stories not only entertain, but also offer practical examples of how to deal with difficult feelings.

Games are also powerful resources to reinforce these teachings. Games that stimulate the repetition of Ho'oponopono phrases, such as the "mirror" game, where the child looks into their own eyes while saying the phrases, help to internalize the concepts of self-love and forgiveness. Another playful activity can be the "cleaning the house" game, where children imagine they are removing invisible dust from a room, symbolizing the cleansing of negative thoughts and feelings. This type of activity makes the process of self-knowledge light and enjoyable.

Drawings and paintings also play an essential role in emotional expression. Encouraging the child to draw situations that made them sad or angry and then using the Ho'oponopono phrases to "cleanse" these feelings promotes emotional release in a creative way. The vibrant colors and free strokes allow children to express their emotions non-verbally, facilitating understanding and acceptance of these experiences. After this process, they can redraw the scene with elements that symbolize love and gratitude, reinforcing the idea of emotional transformation.

Music, in turn, offers an engaging way to reinforce the teachings of Ho'oponopono. Songs that address themes such as forgiveness, love, and gratitude naturally capture children's attention. Musicality not only entertains, but also helps to fix important concepts unconsciously. Singing along with children creates an environment of connection and joy, while positive messages are internalized effortlessly.

The benefits of this practice for child development are broad and profound. On the emotional level, Ho'oponopono helps children understand and deal with their feelings in a healthy way. They learn to identify what they feel, express themselves assertively, and respect their own emotions and those of others. This continuous learning contributes to strengthening self-esteem, allowing them to recognize their intrinsic value and develop self-confidence. When a child understands that they can take care of their emotions and transform them, they feel more secure and capable in the face of everyday challenges.

Interpersonal relationships also benefit from this practice. Ho'oponopono teaches children the importance of empathy, respect, and cooperation. These qualities are essential for building harmonious relationships with family, friends, and colleagues. By understanding that their actions impact others, children become more sensitive to the needs and feelings of those who live with them. This promotes an environment of mutual respect, where communication is more open and conflicts are resolved peacefully.

Speaking of conflicts, Ho'oponopono offers effective tools for children to learn to deal with disagreements maturely. They begin to seek solutions through dialogue and understanding, avoiding impulsive or aggressive reactions. This ability to resolve conflicts serenely is valuable not only in childhood, but throughout life.

Another fundamental aspect that Ho'oponopono develops is personal responsibility. Children begin to realize that they are responsible for their thoughts, feelings, and actions, understanding that they have the power to create their own reality. This sense of responsibility strengthens autonomy and encourages more conscious and balanced attitudes, shaping individuals who are more prepared to face challenges with resilience.

Finally, cultivating inner peace is one of the most valuable gifts that Ho'oponopono offers children. Constant practice helps to calm the mind and heart, providing serenity even in stressful situations. This inner tranquility is reflected in more balanced attitudes, favoring emotional health and general well-being.

By teaching Ho'oponopono to children, we are contributing to forming a generation of agents of transformation. These little ones, by incorporating the practice into their routines, spread seeds of harmony and healing wherever they go. They understand that by taking care of themselves, they also positively influence the environment around them. This virtuous cycle generates lasting impacts, promoting a culture of peace, respect, and compassion.

Therefore, by sowing Ho'oponopono in childhood, we are not only supporting the emotional growth of children, but also collaborating in the construction of a more loving, conscious, and peaceful world. Today's children are the seeds of tomorrow, and by offering them tools to deal with emotions and promote good, we are preparing them to flourish as balanced, resilient adults committed to a better future.

By encouraging the practice of Ho'oponopono from childhood, we open space for children to grow with a deeper understanding of themselves and the world around them. This inner connection strengthens not only how they deal with their own emotions, but also how they interact with the environment, promoting more conscious and empathetic attitudes. With this solid foundation, they will be more prepared to face life's challenges in a balanced and positive way, becoming emotionally healthy and resilient adults.

Furthermore, the involvement of families in this process enhances the benefits of Ho'oponopono, creating more harmonious homes and stronger family relationships. When parents and children share moments of reflection and healing, they strengthen their emotional bonds and build a network of emotional support that favors collective growth. This safe and loving environment encourages open communication and the peaceful resolution of conflicts, contributing to the well-being of all.

By integrating Ho'oponopono into the emotional formation of children, we are planting seeds of love, respect, and responsibility that will flourish throughout their lives. This simple but profoundly transformative practice has the power to shape a more conscious, empathetic generation prepared to transform the world with kindness and wisdom. Thus, each child becomes a light of healing and balance, radiating peace and compassion wherever they go.

# Chapter 17
# Harmony and Healing in the Relationship

Living with pets is a profound experience of emotional and energetic connection, capable of promoting balance and well-being for both humans and animals. These loyal companions are constant sources of affection, joy, and comfort, becoming an essential part of the family environment. In the context of Ho'oponopono, this relationship goes beyond physical care, involving an energetic exchange that reflects our emotional states and behavior patterns. Thus, by taking care of our inner balance, we positively influence the health and behavior of our animals, creating a more harmonious and loving relationship.

Pets have the sensitivity to capture and reflect the emotions of the people they live with, acting as true emotional mirrors. Often, changes in their behavior or health can signal imbalances in the family environment or in the feelings of their guardians. This perception invites us to take responsibility not only for physical care but also for the emotional environment we provide. By practicing Ho'oponopono, we direct intentions of love, forgiveness, and gratitude that help dissolve negative memories and energies, creating a lighter and safer space for our animals.

By integrating Ho'oponopono into our daily lives with our animals, we strengthen bonds of unconditional love and mutual respect. The conscious practice of taking responsibility for one's own emotions, combined with physical and emotional care, contributes to the healing of imbalances and reinforces the harmony of living together. This path of deep connection not only favors the health and happiness of animals but also teaches us about empathy, patience, and the importance of living in the present with lightness. This continuous exchange of love and healing enriches the shared journey, transforming coexistence into an experience of growth and well-being for all.

Living with pets transcends mere physical care and reveals itself as a journey of deep emotional and energetic connection. Our four-legged companions, with their silent and welcoming presence, have the incredible ability to capture and reflect our most subtle emotional states. This natural sensitivity makes them true mirrors of the soul, revealing aspects of ourselves that often remain hidden until they are reflected in their behavior or health. Situations of stress, anxiety, or emotional imbalances in guardians can, for example, manifest themselves in unusual attitudes or even illnesses in animals, signaling the need for attention not only to the physical but also to the shared emotional environment.

By integrating the practice of Ho'oponopono into this relationship, we open the way for deep and mutual healing. This Hawaiian philosophy of reconciliation and forgiveness invites us to look with more responsibility at the reality we co-create with our animals. Every thought, emotion, and action directly influences the environment in which we live and, consequently, impacts those who share that space with us. When we use the simple and powerful words of Ho'oponopono — "I'm sorry. Please forgive me. I love you. I'm grateful." — directed at the memories and emotions that generate imbalances, we are not only promoting our own healing but also contributing to the well-being of our animals.

This process of emotional cleansing begins with the recognition of our responsibility. It is not about guilt, but about understanding that we have the power to transform the energy that circulates in our coexistence. By assuming this posture, we can dissolve memories of difficult moments, such as frustrations, fights, or impatience directed at our animals. With constant practice, we create a lighter, safer, and more loving environment where harmony flourishes naturally. This energetic change directly impacts how animals behave and feel, providing them with a space of welcome and tranquility.

Intuitive communication also plays a fundamental role in this process. Animals have a way of communicating that transcends words. Their looks, gestures, and behaviors are genuine expressions of their needs and emotions. When we allow ourselves to observe carefully and listen with our hearts, we develop a deeper connection, capable of capturing these subtle messages. Ho'oponopono helps us silence mental noise and be truly present, favoring this silent and intuitive dialogue with our animals.

Visualizing our companions healthy, happy, and in harmony is a powerful tool within this practice. By closing our eyes and imagining moments of affection, play, and peace, we are energetically collaborating to create this reality. This visualization, accompanied by the Ho'oponopono phrases, reinforces the intention of healing and balance, projecting love and gratitude for every interaction we have with our animals. This practice not only strengthens the bond but also acts as an energetic balm that soothes tensions and promotes well-being.

Expressing unconditional love is perhaps the most precious lesson that animals teach us daily. They accept us as we are, without judgments or demands. By reciprocating this love genuinely, recognizing their uniqueness, respecting their limits, and taking care of their physical and emotional needs, we create a continuous cycle of affection and healing. This love, free of conditions, is one of the pillars of Ho'oponopono and manifests itself in simple but deeply meaningful gestures, such as a loving look, a caress, or a moment of play.

Physical care, in turn, is an extension of this love. Ensuring adequate nutrition, exercise, hygiene, and regular veterinary follow-up is a concrete way of demonstrating respect and care. However, this care gains an even deeper dimension when carried out with full attention and presence. Each moment of care can be transformed into an opportunity for connection and healing when carried out with loving intention and awareness. Thus, Ho'oponopono invites us to make each interaction an expression of integral care, uniting body, mind, and spirit.

When health or behavioral problems arise, the practice of Ho'oponopono can be a powerful ally to medical treatment. Clearing memories and emotions that may be contributing to the animal's imbalance enhances the healing process. However, it is essential to remember that this practice does not replace veterinary care but complements it, acting on subtle and profound levels. This integral care favors recovery and well-being, promoting harmony in all dimensions of coexistence.

Harmony between species manifests when we recognize that animals are sentient and conscious beings, endowed with their own wisdom. They teach us daily about the importance of the present moment, simplicity, and acceptance. Practicing Ho'oponopono with our animals is a way of honoring this wisdom and reciprocating the unconditional love they offer us. This path of mutual respect leads us to a lighter and more balanced coexistence, where each gesture of care and affection becomes a link of healing and connection.

This process of conscious integration leads us to reflect on the impact of our emotions and actions on the environment around us. By taking care of the well-being of our animals, we are naturally invited to take care of ourselves. Small gestures of attention, presence, and love become powerful agents of transformation, not only in the relationship with our animals but in all areas of our lives. This cycle of balance and well-being expands, positively influencing our family and social relationships and even our bond with nature.

Thus, by deepening this connection with responsibility and love, we create a space where harmony and healing can flourish naturally and continuously. Animals teach us patience, empathy, and the beauty of living with simplicity. By recognizing these teachings and applying them in our daily lives, we not only enrich the relationship with our pets but also transform ourselves. This journey of mutual growth invites us to live with more lightness, compassion, and gratitude, promoting an environment of peace and love that benefits all beings. The relationship with our pets teaches us about unconditional love, loyalty, the joy of living in the present moment, and the importance of connecting with nature. Ho'oponopono invites us to honor this connection between species, recognizing the wisdom and love that animals bring to our lives.

By practicing Ho'oponopono with our pets, we open a channel of mutual healing that transcends words and manifests itself in gestures of affection, presence, and care. This bond teaches us to respect the time and needs of each being, developing in us a more attentive listening and a more compassionate gaze. The harmony resulting from this practice not only strengthens the emotional and physical health of the animals but also allows us to experience a lighter and more balanced coexistence, where love flows naturally and constantly.

This conscious integration also leads us to a broader perception of the impact of our actions on the environment in which we live. Taking care of the well-being of our animals is, at the same time, an invitation to take care of ourselves and the space we share. Small gestures of attention and affection become powerful agents of transformation, creating a continuous cycle of balance and well-being. Thus, the practice of Ho'oponopono extends, positively influencing all relationships around us.

By understanding the depth of this bond, we recognize that living with our animals is a constant exchange of teachings about patience, acceptance, and unconditional love. They show us the value of being present and the beauty of simplicity. By cultivating this connection with responsibility and awareness, we create an environment where harmony flourishes, allowing healing to manifest naturally and lastingly, enriching the shared journey of growth and learning.

# Chapter 18
# Financial Prosperity with Awareness

Financial prosperity is a natural expression of inner balance and harmony with the energy of abundance. When we connect deeply with the flow of life, we recognize that money is an extension of our own vibration and the choices we make daily. It is not just a material resource but a concrete manifestation of our mindset of worthiness, gratitude, and responsibility. By understanding that our relationship with money reflects internal patterns of thought and emotion, it becomes possible to align our energy with prosperity consciously and sustainably. This connection allows us to attract resources with fluidity, manage with wisdom, and share with generosity, creating a virtuous cycle of growth and fulfillment.

Developing a mindset of abundance requires recognizing limiting beliefs that may be blocking the flow of finances. Many of these beliefs are rooted in past experiences, family influences, or social conditioning, which associate money with feelings of guilt, fear, or scarcity. Overcoming these blocks requires a sincere commitment to self-responsibility and self-transformation. By taking control of our financial reality, we open space to reframe old perceptions and create new possibilities. This change in perspective strengthens personal confidence and allows us to use money in a balanced way, as a means to achieve goals and contribute positively to the world around us.

True financial prosperity arises when we use money consciously and purposefully, recognizing its role as a tool for growth and personal fulfillment. By cultivating gratitude for what we already have and adopting conscious financial management practices, we expand our ability to attract and multiply resources. This constant flow of abundance becomes more potent when aligned with actions of generosity and collaboration, strengthening not only our economic stability but also our positive impact on society. Living in harmony with money is, therefore, a path of balance between receiving, managing, and sharing, allowing us to build a full, meaningful life aligned with our deepest values.

Money, far beyond being just a medium of exchange or a material resource, is an energy in constant motion, directly reflecting our thoughts, emotions, and attitudes towards prosperity. From an early age, we are influenced by limiting beliefs that shape our financial perception. These beliefs, often rooted in family or social experiences, associate money with feelings of scarcity, fear, or guilt. This conditioning impedes the natural flow of abundance and restricts our ability to attract and manage resources consciously.

However, Ho'oponopono offers us a path to transform this relationship with money, allowing us to clear memories and beliefs that limit our prosperity. Through the simple and powerful phrases — "I'm sorry.

Please forgive me. I love you. I'm grateful." — we can reprogram our minds, dissolving emotional blocks and opening space for a new financial reality. This process of energetic cleansing not only relieves the burden of negative experiences but also creates conditions for abundance to flow with more lightness and naturalness in our lives.

Taking responsibility for one's own financial reality is the first step in this transformation process. This responsibility does not imply guilt, but rather the recognition that we are co-creators of our experience with money. When we accept this active role, we cease to be victims of circumstances and begin to act consciously, making decisions that favor balance and financial growth. This change in perspective allows us to identify harmful behavior patterns, such as impulsive spending or fear of investing, and replace them with healthier habits aligned with our goals.

Cultivating gratitude for the money we already have, regardless of the amount, is another fundamental practice to attract prosperity. Gratitude connects us with the present abundance and expands our capacity to receive more. By giving thanks for small financial achievements and the opportunities that arise, we send a message of recognition and openness to new possibilities to the universe. This genuine feeling of gratitude strengthens the energetic flow of money, transforming it into an ally in the realization of our dreams.

The practice of visualization also plays an essential role in building a new financial reality.

Imagining yourself living with abundance, fulfilling dreams, investing safely, and contributing to important causes creates a vibration aligned with prosperity. This mental exercise, when performed with regularity and intention, reprograms the subconscious and attracts situations and opportunities that resonate with this new frequency. Visualization, combined with the Ho'oponopono phrases, enhances the creation of a more solid and rewarding financial path.

Furthermore, the use of positive affirmations reinforces this inner transformation. Phrases like "I am worthy of prosperity," "Money flows to me with ease and joy," or "I manage my finances wisely" have the power to replace thoughts of scarcity with ideas of abundance. Repeating these affirmations with conviction helps dissolve limiting patterns and strengthens confidence in one's own ability to attract and maintain financial resources.

However, attracting money is only part of the process. Conscious management of financial resources is fundamental to maintaining and expanding prosperity. This involves planning, organization, and responsible choices. Setting clear goals, controlling expenses, saving, and investing strategically are practices that sustain the continuous flow of abundance. When we align financial care with our intention to prosper, we create a solid foundation for sustainable growth.

Sharing abundance is another essential aspect to keep the financial flow active. Generosity, whether through donations, support for social projects, or helping people close to us, strengthens the cycle of prosperity.

By contributing what we have, we recognize the interconnection between all beings and collaborate to build a more balanced and just world. This act of sharing not only benefits the recipient but also expands our own ability to attract more, as it keeps the flow of giving and receiving in constant motion.

Understanding that money is a tool, not an end in itself, allows us to use it more consciously and aligned with our values. It should be seen as a resource that enhances our achievements and expands our positive impact on the world. When we use it to make dreams come true, support meaningful causes, and provide well-being to ourselves and others, money takes on a transformative role in our lives. This conscious and balanced use reinforces the harmony between material prosperity and personal fulfillment.

By applying Ho'oponopono in the pursuit of financial prosperity, we are invited to reflect on how our thoughts and emotions shape our economic reality. Clearing negative memories and cultivating positive feelings such as gratitude, love, and trust create an energetic foundation conducive to growth. This process not only improves our relationship with money but also leads us to wiser and more responsible decisions, promoting sustainable prosperity aligned with our purposes.

This change in mindset drives us to act with more awareness, choosing investments that resonate with our values and avoiding waste. This new posture strengthens the cycle of abundance, where receiving and sharing balance each other, creating a constant flow of personal and collective growth. True wealth manifests when we prosper financially without losing sight of what truly matters: living with purpose, gratitude, and integrity.

By walking with this new vision of money, we understand that prosperity goes beyond accumulating wealth. It is about using the resources we have wisely and responsibly, creating a full and meaningful life. The balance between achieving financial stability and maintaining connection with our deepest values is what leads us to a harmonious and fulfilling existence.

Thus, Ho'oponopono teaches us that financial prosperity is accessible to all who are willing to clear limiting beliefs and align themselves with the energy of abundance. This path leads us to a lighter and more conscious relationship with money, where each financial choice is guided by gratitude, responsibility, and the genuine desire to contribute positively to the world. By cultivating this new perception, we create not only economic stability but also a life richer in meaning, purpose, and fulfillment.

By integrating Ho'oponopono in the pursuit of financial prosperity, we develop a lighter and healthier relationship with money, recognizing it as a tool that enhances our achievements and expands our positive impact on the world. This practice invites us to release fears and insecurities, replacing them with thoughts of confidence, gratitude, and worthiness. By clearing the memories that feed scarcity, we open space for new financial opportunities to arise naturally, allowing abundance to flow continuously and sustainably in our lives.

This change in perspective also encourages us to act with responsibility and awareness, using our resources in a balanced and strategic way. With a mindset aligned with abundance, we begin to make wiser financial decisions, investing in our dreams and contributing to causes that resonate with our values. This posture strengthens the cycle of prosperity, where the act of receiving and sharing complement each other, creating a harmonious flow of personal and collective growth.

By walking with this new vision of money, we understand that true wealth lies in living according to our purpose, enjoying material achievements without distancing ourselves from our essence. The balance between prospering financially and maintaining connection with our deepest values leads us to a full life, where each choice is guided by awareness, gratitude, and the genuine desire to contribute to a more abundant and harmonious world.

# Chapter 19
# Home Purification

The home represents a sacred space of welcome, balance, and renewal, where every detail directly influences the physical, emotional, and spiritual well-being of those who inhabit it. More than walls and objects, it carries the energy of lived experiences, shared emotions, and intentions deposited in each environment. The harmony of the home reflects the care taken with the space and, above all, the inner balance of its residents. Recognizing the importance of this environment, it becomes essential to keep its energy clean and light, creating a haven of peace that promotes emotional, mental, and spiritual health.

Each room, object, and corner of the house carries memories and vibrations that can positively or negatively impact family dynamics and emotional state. Disorganized environments or those overloaded with unnecessary objects accumulate not only dust but also stagnant energies that can generate discomfort, tiredness, and even conflicts. The purification of the home involves a conscious connection with this space, promoting its physical and energetic cleansing. This process allows vital energy to circulate freely, creating a lighter, more inspiring, and welcoming environment that strengthens the connection with one's own essence and with those who share the same space.

Caring for the home with love and intention is a transformative practice that goes beyond organization and aesthetics. It is about nourishing the environment with gratitude, light, and harmony, allowing it to become a true refuge of serenity and renewal. Small gestures, such as opening windows to allow the entry of fresh air and natural light, cultivating plants that bring life and purify the air, or using soft aromas that elevate the vibration of the environment, contribute to creating a balanced and energized space. This conscious care transforms the home into a place conducive to rest, creativity, harmonious coexistence, and the manifestation of a full and happy life.

Just as the physical body reflects our emotional and mental state, the home directly manifests the quality of our emotions, thoughts, and experiences. Each environment in the house holds energetic impressions that can influence mood, health, and even relationships between residents. A disorganized space, loaded with purposeless objects or neglected in its cleanliness, accumulates not only dust but also stagnant energies. This accumulation creates a dense atmosphere that can generate discomfort, tiredness, and even conflicts, affecting emotional balance and family harmony. Therefore, the purification of the home becomes essential, not only as a practice of physical cleaning but as a true ritual of energetic and spiritual renewal.

Ho'oponopono offers us a profound approach to this purification. The Hawaiian philosophy, centered on forgiveness and reconciliation, teaches us that everything around us is a reflection of what we carry within. Thus, when we direct the phrases "I'm sorry. Please forgive me. I love you. I'm grateful." to the environments of our home, we are cleaning not only the energy of the physical space but also the emotional memories associated with it. Each room, object, and corner of the house is recognized as an integral part of our history and, therefore, deserves care, respect, and love. This conscious process creates a lighter, more inspiring, and welcoming atmosphere.

Purification begins with physical cleaning. Organizing the space, eliminating objects that no longer have a purpose, and keeping the house clean are essential steps to release energy flow. The accumulation of purposeless objects represents stagnation, and by detaching ourselves from what no longer serves us, we open space for new energies and opportunities. This material detachment directly reflects on the emotional, relieving the weight of past memories and allowing vital energy to circulate freely throughout the environment.

Energy cleansing complements this process. In addition to Ho'oponopono, practices such as the use of incense, smudging, or herbal sprays help dissolve dense vibrations. Directing the Ho'oponopono phrases to each environment enhances purification, transforming the space into a haven of peace. Visualizing a soft light filling each room while repeating the healing words contributes to the creation of a serene and balanced environment. This practice, done regularly, keeps the vibration of the house elevated and protected from negative energies.

Natural elements also play a fundamental role in harmonizing the home. Plants, for example, are excellent natural purifiers. They revitalize the environment, bring life, balance energies, and contribute to a feeling of freshness and vitality. Having plants at home not only improves air quality but also creates a connection with nature, bringing calm and serenity to the space. Each leaf, each flower, is a reminder of the importance of the cycle of life and constant care.

Natural ventilation is another crucial aspect. Keeping the windows open, allowing the entry of fresh air and sunlight, renews energies and dissipates stagnant vibrations. Sunlight, with its vital energy, is a powerful agent of purification and renewal. It illuminates not only the physical space but also the emotional, bringing clarity, disposition, and well-being. Air circulation promotes energy fluidity, creating a light and welcoming atmosphere.

Music is another powerful tool to raise the vibration of the environment. Soft sounds, mantras, instrumental music, or songs that evoke positive feelings can transform the energy of the space. Sound vibration penetrates walls, objects, and bodies, dissipating tensions and bringing harmony. Incorporating music into the daily life of the home is an invitation for joy, calm, and love to become constant presences in the home.

Crystals are also valuable allies in harmonizing the home. Each crystal carries specific properties that aid in purification and energy balance. Amethyst, for example, promotes peace and tranquility, while black tourmaline protects against negative energies. Positioning crystals at strategic points in the house enhances protection and harmony, creating an energy shield that keeps the environment light and safe.

The practice of gratitude completes this purification process. Thanking for the home, for each room, for each object that serves us in our daily lives, is a way of recognizing the importance of this space in our lives. Gratitude transforms the way we look at the environment, awakening the desire to care for, preserve, and value every detail. When we give thanks, we nourish the space with love and recognition, strengthening the connection with the home as a sacred place.

This conscious care for the physical and energetic environment of the home directly reflects family relationships and quality of life. A clean and harmonized space favors dialogue, mutual understanding, and peaceful coexistence. Conflicts dissolve more easily in an environment where lightness and harmony reign. The home becomes a true sanctuary where each family member finds welcome, security, and inspiration to live in balance.

By recognizing the home as an extension of our inner world, we understand that each gesture of care reverberates positively in our physical, emotional, and spiritual health. Caring for the space in which we live is, above all, caring for ourselves. This process of attention and affection for the environment strengthens us in the face of daily challenges, offering a safe haven for rest, introspection, and the renewal of energies.

Transforming the home into a space of balance does not require major changes, but rather small actions carried out with intention. Opening the windows every morning, lighting incense at the end of the day, caring for plants, reorganizing a corner of the house, or simply stopping to give thanks for this space are attitudes that, when added together, create an environment of peace and prosperity. These practices teach us the importance of the present, to value what we have, and to cultivate serenity in small things.

When we understand that the environment around us profoundly influences our internal state, we begin to see the home with different eyes. Each room becomes a reflection of our journey, a space for learning and healing. The house ceases to be just a physical shelter and transforms into a sacred space where the energy of peace, love, and abundance flows freely, nourishing body, mind, and spirit.

Thus, by integrating Ho'oponopono and purification practices into home care, we create a harmonious and revitalizing environment. This space becomes more than just a place to rest; it becomes a true temple of balance, renewal, and love. Every detail, every gesture of care, strengthens this sacred bond between us and our home, allowing the energy of healing and serenity to fully manifest in our lives.

By caring for the home with intention and presence, we create a space where energy flows lightly and harmoniously, promoting the well-being of all who live there. Each gesture of care, from physical cleaning to energy purification, reinforces the bond between the environment and our essence. Thus, the home ceases to be just a place of rest and transforms into a true sanctuary of balance and renewal, capable of strengthening us in the face of daily challenges and inspiring us to live with more lightness and gratitude.

This harmony cultivated in the environment directly reflects family relationships and daily interactions. A purified and energized home becomes fertile ground for dialogue, understanding, and emotional connection. Ho'oponopono practices, when applied frequently, dissolve accumulated tensions and promote an atmosphere of peace and welcome. This safe and loving space allows us to freely express who we are, strengthen emotional bonds, and nurture moments of joy and complicity.

By recognizing the home as an extension of our inner world, we realize that every detail, no matter how small, contributes to the construction of an environment of harmony and prosperity. This awareness invites us to care for our space with love, respect, and gratitude, creating a refuge where the energy of peace, abundance, and love can flow freely. Thus, we live in a home that not only shelters us but also welcomes, inspires, and heals us, becoming an essential part of our journey of evolution and balance.

# Chapter 20
# Messages from the Subconscious

Dreams reveal deep aspects of our mind, functioning as direct channels of communication from the subconscious. They expose hidden emotions, thoughts, and memories, offering valuable clues about internal issues that need attention and healing. In Ho'oponopono, these dream signs are recognized as manifestations of memories that need to be cleansed, unresolved conflicts, and necessary learning. Careful analysis of these messages allows access to essential information for self-knowledge and the process of inner transformation. Each symbolic or emotional detail present in dreams carries a unique meaning, which can guide the individual on their journey of healing and emotional balance.

By understanding dreams from the perspective of Ho'oponopono, it is possible to realize that they are not merely random manifestations of the mind, but direct reflections of past experiences and repressed emotions. These contents emerge during sleep when the conscious mind is quiet and the subconscious gains space to express itself. This process reveals behavior patterns, limiting beliefs, and painful memories that influence daily choices and attitudes. Recognizing these signs with clarity and willingness to interpret them opens paths to deep emotional cleansing, allowing internal blocks to be dissolved with compassion and self-love.

Integrating the practice of observing and interpreting dreams into the Ho'oponopono cleansing process strengthens the bond with inner wisdom. Keeping a dream journal, reflecting on recurring symbols, and applying the purification phrases contribute to releasing accumulated emotions and restoring emotional balance. This continuous process promotes self-knowledge and facilitates connection with the divine essence, allowing each dream experience to be used as a tool for growth and healing. Thus, dreams become precious guides, guiding the way to a lighter, more conscious, and harmonious life.

Dreams are silent portals that connect us to the deepest layers of the subconscious, revealing emotions, thoughts, and memories that often remain hidden during the waking state. In this dream universe, symbols, metaphors, and archetypes emerge as subtle languages that reflect our inner conflicts, our limiting beliefs, and the memories that need to be understood and healed. In the context of Ho'oponopono, these dreams are not seen as mere random manifestations of the mind, but as clear signs of internal aspects that require attention, love, and transmutation. Each detail, each sensation experienced during sleep carries a unique meaning, an invitation to self-knowledge and the release of emotional blocks.

When we fall asleep, the conscious mind withdraws, and the subconscious takes control. It is at this moment that repressed emotions, unresolved traumas, and deeply rooted behavior patterns have space to emerge, often through symbols that escape rational logic. These signs, however confusing or disconnected they may seem, are valuable clues to parts of us that still need to be embraced. Recognizing this communication is essential so that we can begin a healing process. Ho'oponopono guides us to see these dream fragments as reflections of memories that ask to be cleansed, understood, and transformed.

Keeping a dream journal is a powerful practice on this path of self-knowledge. Writing down immediately upon awakening all the details and emotions felt in dreams allows access to deep layers of the subconscious mind. It is not just about recording images or events, but about diving into the sensations that each dream evokes. This constant exercise of observation creates a bridge between the conscious and the subconscious, allowing hidden patterns to become clearer and more understandable. The act of writing then becomes a form of dialogue with forgotten or neglected internal parts.

In addition to recording, careful observation of the symbols present in dreams plays a fundamental role in this process. Although some symbols have universal meanings, such as water representing emotions or flying symbolizing freedom, the true meaning of each image is deeply linked to individual experience and perception. Thus, interpreting dreams requires sensitivity to perceive what each symbol represents personally. Ho'oponopono invites us to approach this interpretation with love and compassion, without judgment, recognizing that each dream element has something to teach or heal.

The emotions felt during the dream are even more revealing than the symbols themselves. Fear, joy, anger, or serenity experienced in this state reveal emotional states that are often not fully recognized in everyday life. Observing these emotions and relating them to current or past experiences brings clarity about what needs to be embraced and transformed. Ho'oponopono, in this context, becomes an essential tool. By directing its purification phrases — "I'm sorry. Please forgive me. I love you. I'm grateful." — to these emotions and symbols that emerge, the process of cleansing and releasing these memories begins.

Establishing a direct dialogue with the subconscious before sleep is also a transformative practice. When lying down, it is possible to make a clear intention: ask the subconscious to reveal, through dreams, what needs to be understood and healed. This request opens space for more conscious and fluid communication with internal content. Likewise, upon awakening, it is possible to give thanks for the messages received, even if they are not yet fully understood, trusting that, in time, clarity will emerge.

Memory cleansing associated with dreams is a delicate but profoundly liberating step. Directing the Ho'oponopono phrases to the characters, situations, and feelings that arise in dreams is a way to dissolve dense energies and transform limiting patterns. By repeating "I'm sorry. Please forgive me. I love you. I'm grateful," we are recognizing that something within us needs to be healed, taking responsibility for these contents and allowing the inner divinity to transmute these memories.

Dreams can also be powerful guides for decisions and changes in various areas of life. They can alert us to behaviors that need to be adjusted, beliefs that limit growth, or even suggest paths that favor personal and spiritual development. When we look at dreams with attention and wisdom, they cease to be just disconnected images and become compasses that guide us towards fulfillment and balance.

Over time, this continuous practice of observing, recording, interpreting, and cleansing memories brought by dreams strengthens the connection with one's own intuition. Trust in one's own inner wisdom deepens, and sensitivity to perceiving emotional nuances expands. Dreams come to be recognized not only as reflections of past issues but as opportunities for learning, growth, and renewal.

This integration between the dream world and the conscious practice of Ho'oponopono leads to a continuous process of healing and transformation. By embracing dream messages with compassion and applying the emotional cleansing proposed by Ho'oponopono, we gently dissolve internal blocks, allowing peace and balance to settle in naturally. This process does not require haste or immediate answers, but rather presence, patience, and openness to listen to what the soul has to say.

With each dream understood and each memory cleansed, the individual moves forward with more lightness on their journey. Clarity emerges, and with it comes the ability to deal with daily challenges in a more serene and conscious way. The harmony between the inner and outer world is strengthened, creating a state of balance that reverberates positively in all areas of life.

Thus, by recognizing dreams as allies in the process of self-knowledge, each nocturnal experience is transformed into an opportunity for healing and growth. Ho'oponopono, when integrated into this practice, promotes deep emotional release, allowing life to flow with more lightness, clarity, and purpose. In this way, we continue on our journey more connected with our essence, guided by an inner wisdom that guides us with love and compassion towards wholeness.

This journey of self-discovery through dreams reveals itself as a constant invitation to inner reconciliation. Each symbol unveiled and each emotion understood become fundamental pieces in the healing process, allowing memories to be gently transmuted. By applying Ho'oponopono practices in this context, a safe space is created to embrace repressed feelings and dissolve emotional blocks, promoting harmony that reverberates in all aspects of life.

Over time, this integration between the dream world and the conscious practice of emotional cleansing strengthens trust in one's own intuition. Dreams come to be recognized not only as reflections of the past but as wise messages that indicate new possibilities for growth. This constant dialogue with the subconscious develops a keener perception of inner needs and awakens a sensitivity to deal with daily challenges in a lighter and more compassionate way.

Thus, by embracing dreams as allies on the path of self-knowledge, each nocturnal experience is transformed into an opportunity for renewal. The continuous practice of Ho'oponopono in the face of these subtle messages promotes a profound inner liberation, allowing peace and balance to settle in naturally. In this way, the individual advances on their journey with more clarity and serenity, aligned with their essence and open to the infinite possibilities of healing and transformation.

# Chapter 21
# Aging with Wisdom and Serenity

Aging represents a valuable stage of existence, full of opportunities to deepen the connection with oneself and the world around. Far from being a period of loss, this phase offers the chance to cultivate a deeper wisdom, reframe past experiences, and live with more lightness and authenticity. As the body undergoes natural transformations, the mind and spirit can flourish, allowing each individual to recognize the importance of caring not only for physical health, but also for emotional and spiritual balance. Ho'oponopono emerges as a powerful practice to navigate this journey with serenity, promoting self-knowledge, acceptance, and gratitude for each experience lived.

Embracing the aging process with wisdom requires a shift in perspective, moving away from the negative view often imposed by society and recognizing the value of experiences accumulated over time. This period of life provides the chance to strengthen inner resilience and transform challenges into opportunities for growth. Self-care and reflection practices, such as Ho'oponopono, encourage the release of limiting beliefs and cultivate a harmonious relationship with one's own body and mind. Thus, each moment is lived with more meaning, allowing maturity to transform into a state of fullness and peace.

By understanding aging as a natural and enriching cycle, space is opened for a more conscious and intentional experience. The accumulated experience becomes an inexhaustible source of learning and inspiration, not only for oneself but also for future generations. Living this phase with purpose and enthusiasm means valuing each achievement, nurturing meaningful relationships, and keeping the pursuit of new knowledge alive. In this way, maturity is revealed as a period of inner expansion, where serenity and wisdom guide each step with confidence and gratitude.

1. Aging: A New Phase of the Journey

Aging is a natural and inevitable process, marked by physical, mental, and emotional changes. Western society, with its emphasis on youth and external beauty, often associates aging with decline and loss. However, Ho'oponopono invites us to reframe this perception, recognizing aging as an opportunity for growth, wisdom, and self-knowledge.

Aging with health and vitality is a deep desire of many, but not always fully understood. Ho'oponopono emerges as an invitation to care not only for the physical body, but also for the mind and spirit, providing balance in all dimensions of existence. Accepting aging as a natural part of life is the first step in navigating this journey with lightness. When one recognizes that physical transformations are inevitable, but do not define the totality of being, space is opened for genuine acceptance. This acceptance dissolves internal resistance and frees the individual from the suffering caused by unrealistic expectations, allowing inner peace to be established naturally.

Gratitude then becomes an essential pillar on this path. Valuing each phase lived, each experience accumulated, and each lesson learned transforms the way one views the passing of years. This recognition of the abundance that permeates life generates a deep connection with the present and brings with it a serene joy. Simple moments become more valuable, and relationships become more authentic. Gratitude not only warms the heart but also vitalizes the body, promoting a feeling of continuous well-being.

Self-care manifests as a concrete expression of this love for oneself. Adopting practices that promote physical health, such as a balanced diet, regular exercise, and adequate rest, is essential. However, taking care of the mind and emotions is equally important. Taking time to relax, meditate, and reflect strengthens inner balance and prepares the body to age with dignity. This integral care is a way of honoring one's own body, recognizing it as the temple that sustains all of life's experiences.

Within this process, memory cleansing plays a transformative role. The four phrases of Ho'oponopono — "I'm sorry. Please forgive me. I love you. I'm grateful." — act as powerful tools to free the individual from limiting beliefs surrounding aging. Deeply rooted fears, such as the fear of getting sick, losing autonomy, or facing loneliness, can be softened when these phrases are consciously applied to the memories that sustain them. This process of inner purification paves the way for a new perspective on old age, allowing it to be seen as a time of fullness and not decline.

Positive visualization also contributes to shaping a healthier aging experience. Imagining yourself living with health, joy, and energy renews daily motivation. Visualizing yourself actively participating in life, surrounded by love and wisdom, reinforces the belief that it is possible to live well at any age. This practice strengthens the mind, stimulates hope, and guides daily actions towards choices that favor well-being.

Furthermore, the connection with inner wisdom becomes an inexhaustible source of comfort and guidance. Over the years, the baggage of lived experiences is transformed into a true treasure. Recognizing and valuing this accumulated wisdom allows one not only to face challenges with more confidence, but also to share this knowledge with younger generations. This gesture of transmitting knowledge not only strengthens family and community ties, but also perpetuates teachings that can positively impact the lives of many.

Aging with purpose is a proposition that transcends the simple passage of time. Ho'oponopono invites us to look at each phase of life with gratitude and enthusiasm, recognizing the unique value of each stage. It is not about fighting against time, but about embracing it, taking advantage of the opportunities it offers to grow, learn, and contribute. Continuing to learn, developing new skills, and sharing experiences enriches the journey and keeps the flame of curiosity and passion for life alive.

This perspective of purpose is reflected in small and large daily actions. Seeking new experiences, staying open to change, and cultivating healthy relationships are ways to nurture the spirit. Actively participating in the community, getting involved in social causes, or simply being present to listen and advise make aging a phase of great contribution to the world. It is in this continuous learning and sharing that the true meaning of aging with purpose is found.

Celebrating life in all its stages is another valuable lesson that Ho'oponopono teaches. Each phase — childhood, youth, adulthood, and old age — has its own beauty and challenges. Recognizing and honoring each of these phases as essential parts of a rich and unique story allows one to live with more fullness. Old age, then, is no longer seen as an end but is understood as an expansion of existence, a period where one can reap the fruits of what has been sown throughout life.

This continuous celebration of life translates into a loving acceptance of each memory, each change, and each emotion. By practicing Ho'oponopono, an inner space of serenity is created, where unrealistic expectations are dissolved and replaced by a compassionate understanding of oneself and the natural cycle of life. This state of full presence provides a lightness that makes aging more fluid and natural.

Sharing the wisdom acquired over the years is not only an act of generosity, but a powerful form of connection with future generations. When experiences and learning are transmitted with love, they have the power to inspire, guide, and strengthen those who are beginning to tread their own paths. This continuous flow of learning creates support networks that benefit both those who teach and those who learn, weaving a web of affection and solidarity.

With this broader and more welcoming view, aging is revealed as a period full of meaning and purpose. The constant practice of Ho'oponopono strengthens inner peace, deepens gratitude, and brings lightness to the journey, allowing each moment to be lived with fullness. Thus, maturity becomes a fertile field for inner renewal, where serenity guides each step and wisdom illuminates the path. In this harmonious flow of acceptance and love, life unfolds in its entirety, rich in harmony and deeply connected with what truly matters.

This continuous celebration of life allows aging to be seen as an expansion of existence itself, where each lived experience is transformed into a solid foundation for new discoveries. By practicing Ho'oponopono, the individual learns to embrace each memory, each change, and each emotion with love, creating an inner space of acceptance and serenity. This state of full presence facilitates the detachment from unrealistic expectations and promotes a more compassionate understanding of oneself and the natural cycle of life.

Sharing the wisdom acquired over the years also becomes a powerful way to connect with future generations. Knowledge transmitted with love and generosity inspires and guides those who are beginning their own journeys. This flow of continuous learning strengthens family and community ties, creating support networks that nurture both those who teach and those who learn. Thus, aging is not just an individual process, but an opportunity to contribute to collective growth.

With this broader and more welcoming perspective, aging is revealed as a phase full of meaning and purpose. By integrating Ho'oponopono into daily routine, peace, gratitude, and lightness are cultivated, allowing each moment to be lived with fullness. In this way, maturity becomes a fertile space for inner renewal, where serenity guides each step and wisdom illuminates the path, leading to a life rich in harmony and love.

# Chapter 22
# Finding Relief and Healing

Pain, in its many forms, appears as a clear sign that something in our body or mind requires attention and care. This experience, although challenging, carries with it the possibility of healing and profound transformation. Facing pain with awareness allows us to identify its roots and understand that it does not have to be a permanent burden, but rather a starting point for self-knowledge and overcoming. Ho'oponopono offers an effective way to deal with this suffering, promoting the release of memories and beliefs that intensify pain and opening space for relief and inner balance.

By recognizing pain as a natural part of existence, it is possible to develop a more compassionate relationship with oneself, welcoming emotions and sensations without resistance. This process involves not only accepting vulnerability, but also seeking to understand the internal causes that fuel discomfort. Through the constant practice of Ho'oponopono, it becomes feasible to dissolve limiting patterns, soften the impact of painful experiences, and allow the energy of healing to flow freely. This approach brings relief and strengthens the ability to face challenges with serenity and confidence.

The journey to healing requires openness and willingness to transform pain into learning. By adopting practices such as acceptance, compassion, and memory cleansing, an internal environment conducive to emotional and physical recovery is created. Ho'oponopono encourages the practice of forgiveness and gratitude, essential elements to alleviate suffering and restore harmony. This process not only lessens pain, but also leads to a state of lasting peace, where each experience contributes to personal evolution and complete well-being.

Pain, in its various manifestations, arises as a silent messenger, a reminder that there are internal aspects that cry out for attention and care. It should not be seen only as a nuisance to be eliminated, but as a valuable opportunity to look within and understand what needs to be healed. Physical pain can point to imbalances in the body, while emotional pain often reveals old wounds, limiting beliefs, or disharmonious relationships that remain unresolved. Ho'oponopono invites us not to ignore or suppress these pains, but to embrace them with compassion and understanding. By investigating their origin, it becomes possible to identify memories and patterns that feed suffering, allowing them to be released, paving the way for true healing.

In this process, acceptance plays a fundamental role. Facing pain with courage and serenity, without resistance or judgment, is the first step in dissolving suffering. Acceptance does not mean resignation, but rather the willingness to recognize pain as part of the human experience. This recognition opens space for relief and inner transformation. When we stop fighting against pain, we begin a lighter and more conscious journey of healing.

Compassion for oneself also becomes essential on this path. Many times, we are hard on ourselves in the face of difficulties, demanding strength where it would be more necessary to offer care. Cultivating compassion is allowing yourself to be vulnerable, welcoming yourself with love and respecting your own healing time. This loving gaze softens pain and strengthens the spirit, making the overcoming process more gentle and effective.

The practice of Ho'oponopono is especially powerful in this context. Its four phrases — "I'm sorry. Please forgive me. I love you. I'm grateful." — function as keys to unlock repressed emotions and dissolve memories that feed pain. By directing these words with intention to the pain itself, to the experiences that triggered it, or to the feelings that accompany it, a process of inner cleansing begins. This symbolic and profound act allows old grudges and limiting beliefs to be released, creating a lighter inner space conducive to healing.

Visualizing pain dissipating is also an effective practice. Imagining pain transforming into light, being dissolved and replaced by feelings of peace and well-being, reinforces the power of the mind over the body. This visualization activates the flow of positive energy, contributing to relief and renewing the hope that healing is possible. The energy of healing spreads, involving body and mind, and restores the balance needed to move forward.

Conscious breathing emerges as a simple but powerful tool to alleviate suffering. By breathing slowly and deeply, the mind calms and the body relaxes. This state of serenity reduces the tension that often intensifies pain and allows vital energy to circulate freely. Each conscious breath is an invitation to return to the present and find a point of balance in the midst of discomfort.

Even in times of pain, gratitude can be cultivated. Finding reasons to be thankful, even in the face of suffering, may seem challenging, but this exercise transforms perspective. Gratitude connects us to the abundance of life and strengthens our resilience. Recognizing small moments of relief, the support of loved ones, or the simple ability to breathe can bring comfort and renew hope.

When it comes to physical pain, Ho'oponopono can act as a valuable complement to conventional medical treatments. By clearing memories and beliefs related to illness or injury, we contribute to a more harmonious recovery process. However, it is essential to seek appropriate medical guidance to diagnose and treat the physical causes of pain. Ho'oponopono, in this context, assists in the emotional and energetic dimension of healing, offering support to traditional treatment.

Emotional pain, in turn, is often more complex and silent. Feelings of sadness, anger, fear, or anxiety can become deeply rooted, making them difficult to understand and overcome. The practice of

Ho'oponopono invites you to look at these emotions with compassion, recognizing them as opportunities for self-knowledge. By clearing memories that sustain these emotions, we pave the way to release repressed emotional pain and heal wounds from the past. This process not only relieves emotional weight, but also promotes a feeling of lightness and freedom.

Transcending pain is more than overcoming it — it is transforming it into learning and growth. Ho'oponopono teaches that pain, however uncomfortable it may be, can become a teacher, guiding us to a deeper understanding of ourselves. This path does not require haste, but patience and surrender. Healing does not follow a straight line; there are advances and setbacks, moments of relief and introspection. Respecting this natural rhythm is essential to integrate changes in a lasting way.

By treading this path with awareness, pain ceases to be an obstacle and becomes a portal to self-knowledge. Suffering is transformed into opportunity, and each challenge overcome strengthens confidence in one's own ability to overcome. The constant practice of Ho'oponopono allows us to dissolve the layers of pain accumulated over time, replacing them with feelings of love, gratitude, and peace. This state of inner harmony does not mean the total absence of pain, but rather the presence of a serenity that softens any discomfort.

In this process, self-love is revealed as the basis of transformation. By nurturing this love for oneself, an internal environment is created where healing can flourish naturally. Pain loses its strength when it is embraced with understanding and dissolved with kindness. Thus, the healing journey becomes a path of renewal and growth, where each step is guided by inner wisdom.

Upon reaching this state of fullness, one understands that true healing is not just the elimination of pain, but the integration of all lived experiences. Healing is the full presence of love, gratitude, and balance. It is living with lightness and purpose, recognizing that each challenge overcome shapes a more resilient and conscious being. With Ho'oponopono as an ally, pain dissolves, and a new chapter of peace and renewal begins, leading to a more authentic and harmonious life.

This process of transcendence does not mean denying or minimizing pain, but integrating it as an essential part of the journey. Each discomfort carries within it a valuable message, and by listening carefully to these signs, we can direct our actions towards true healing. Ho'oponopono acts as a bridge between pain and wisdom, gently guiding us to release what no longer serves us and embrace new perspectives of balance and well-being. This path is an invitation to trust in one's own capacity for regeneration and allow self-love to be the basis for transformation.

As we delve deeper into this practice, we realize that healing does not occur in a linear fashion. There are moments of progress and pause, both equally important. Respecting this rhythm is essential to consolidate lasting changes. Ho'oponopono reminds us to be patient with ourselves, understanding that each step taken towards pain relief contributes to building a state of inner serenity. Thus, the healing journey becomes lighter and more conscious, allowing peace to gradually flourish.

With this expanded understanding, pain ceases to be an obstacle and becomes a portal to self-knowledge. By practicing Ho'oponopono with sincerity and constancy, we open space for harmony to be established in all areas of life. Healing, then, is not just the absence of suffering, but the full presence of love, gratitude, and balance. In this state of fullness, we are able to embrace life with more lightness and purpose, ending the cycle of pain and beginning a new chapter of peace and renewal.

# Chapter 23
# Transforming the Energy of Fire

Anger manifests as an intense and instinctive force, capable of awakening deep and immediate reactions. This energy, when understood and directed consciously, reveals itself as a valuable resource for personal growth and inner transformation. In the context of Ho'oponopono, this emotion is not considered an obstacle to be avoided, but a legitimate expression of the human experience that carries an important message. Recognizing anger as an opportunity for self-knowledge and healing allows it to be used constructively, opening space for significant changes in the way we relate to ourselves and others.

Understanding anger involves realizing that it arises as an alert to situations that threaten our values, limits, or expectations. This perception invites us to reflect on the origins of this emotion, identifying memories and beliefs that may be rooted in past experiences. By embracing anger without judgment, it becomes possible to access deeper layers of consciousness, where emotional patterns that influence our reactions are stored. Thus, Ho'oponopono emerges as an effective practice to dissolve these blockages, favoring the release of resentment and the restoration of emotional balance.

Channeling anger in a positive way demands courage and presence. When this energy is transformed, it drives assertive actions, encourages the search for solutions, and strengthens the ability to establish healthy boundaries. This process does not mean suppressing or denying anger, but allowing it to be felt, understood, and transmuted into creative force. From this perspective, anger ceases to be an uncontrolled flame and becomes a fire that illuminates the path to self-awareness, emotional responsibility, and the construction of more authentic and harmonious relationships.

Anger, often seen as a negative and unwanted emotion, is actually a legitimate and powerful expression of the human experience. It arises as an emotional alarm, signaling that our limits have been crossed, our values disrespected, or our expectations frustrated. This inner fire, when understood and embraced with awareness, has the potential to transform into a creative and transformative force. In the context of Ho'oponopono, anger is not seen as something to be repressed or denied, but as an opportunity for self-knowledge and healing. It is through this deeper look that we can use this intense energy constructively, directing it towards creating positive change and strengthening emotional balance.

Understanding the nature of anger requires a careful and conscious approach. This emotion does not arise without reason; it is the result of internal and external triggers that are often rooted in past memories and limiting beliefs. When we identify these triggers, we can realize that many angry reactions are not just related to the present, but are echoes of unresolved experiences. Ho'oponopono offers a profound practice to access these hidden layers of the mind, allowing old emotional patterns to be dissolved. By embracing anger without judgment, we become able to recognize its roots and begin the process of cleansing and releasing these memories that imprison us.

Transforming the energy of anger into something positive requires courage to look inward and responsibility to act consciously. This process begins with careful observation of this emotion. When anger arises, it is essential to pause and reflect: What exactly triggered this feeling? What thoughts accompany it? How does it manifest physically in my body? This exercise in self-perception takes us away from automatic reactions and brings us closer to a clearer understanding of what is really happening within us. From this clarity, we can consciously decide how to deal with this energy in a healthy way.

Taking responsibility for one's own anger is not an act of guilt, but of empowerment. Recognizing that we are the creators of our emotional responses gives us back the power to choose how to react to situations that challenge us. This does not mean accepting disrespectful behavior or injustices, but understanding that we can choose the most assertive and respectful way to express our feelings and set limits. Ho'oponopono reminds us that we have the power to transform anger, not to be controlled by it.

The practice of the four phrases of Ho'oponopono—"I'm sorry. Please forgive me. I love you. I'm grateful."—is a powerful tool to initiate this transformation. By directing these words to the situations that caused the anger, to the people involved, or even to ourselves, we begin to cleanse the memories and negative emotions that fuel this feeling. This process does not erase what happened, but releases the associated emotional weight, allowing us to act with more clarity and serenity.

Expressing anger in a healthy way is another essential step on this journey. Instead of repressing it or exploding it in an uncontrolled way, we can channel it through assertive dialogues, physical activities, or creative practices, such as writing or art. These forms of expression not only release accumulated energy, but also create opportunities to resolve conflicts constructively. Anger, when expressed with respect and awareness, can become a bridge to understanding and problem solving.

Compassion is a powerful ally in this process. Cultivating compassion for yourself allows you to understand that feeling angry does not make you a bad or weak person, but a human one. Similarly, extending this compassion to others helps us to see beyond the actions that hurt us. Often, those who cause us pain are also dealing with their own inner battles. This understanding does not justify harmful behaviors, but dissolves resentment and opens space for forgiveness. Forgiveness, in this context, is an act of liberation—not for the other, but for ourselves. Releasing anger is a gift we give to our own hearts, allowing them to heal and move on in peace.

Transforming the energy of fire that anger represents is like learning to tame an intense flame. It is not about extinguishing it, but about using it to illuminate our paths and warm our intentions. When channeled consciously, this energy drives change, motivates us to act and defend our rights with respect and firmness. Ho'oponopono teaches us to transmute this force into something constructive, helping us to seek solutions and build fairer and more harmonious relationships.

With the continuous practice of Ho'oponopono, we cultivate an inner peace that allows us to deal with anger in a more balanced way. Observing this emotion with awareness, taking responsibility for our reactions, and cleansing the memories that feed it are fundamental steps to finding serenity even in the most challenging moments. This path of self-transformation teaches us that anger can be a powerful ally when understood and directed wisely.

This process, however, is continuous and requires patience. The transformation of anger does not occur immediately, but gradually, as we develop a more conscious relationship with our emotions. Each challenging situation becomes an opportunity for learning and growth. Instead of reacting impulsively, we begin to act with purpose, setting healthy boundaries and expressing our needs clearly and respectfully.

Thus, anger ceases to be seen as an obstacle and becomes recognized as a force that can drive positive change. When we choose to embrace and transmute this emotion with awareness, we open space for a lighter and fuller life. The energy previously consumed by resentment and excessive reactions is transformed into fuel for personal evolution and the construction of more authentic and harmonious relationships.

Thus, transforming the energy of fire does not mean suffocating it, but allowing it to illuminate and warm our path. By practicing Ho'oponopono sincerely, we find a new way to deal with anger—not as an enemy, but as an ally that, when understood, guides us to a more balanced and conscious life. In this process of transmutation, we cultivate serenity, strengthen our bonds, and build a path where inner peace and emotional clarity become pillars for a more authentic and fulfilling existence.

This path of self-understanding and transformation is not built overnight, but requires constant practice and patience. When we realize that anger is just a superficial layer of deeper emotions, we are invited to delve into the roots of these feelings and dissolve old patterns that no longer serve our growth. Ho'oponopono thus becomes a powerful tool for this journey, allowing the energy previously consumed by anger to be directed towards creating more positive and conscious experiences.

Over time, this practice teaches us that each emotion has its purpose and that even anger can be an ally when understood and integrated. Instead of reacting impulsively, we learn to act with clarity and purpose, recognizing our limits and expressing our needs with respect. This balance between feeling and acting strengthens not only our relationship with ourselves, but also with those around us, promoting more authentic and harmonious interactions.

Thus, transforming the energy of fire does not mean extinguishing it, but using it to illuminate our paths and fuel the flame of positive change. When we choose to embrace and transmute anger with awareness and love, we open space for a lighter and fuller life, where each challenge is seen as an opportunity for evolution. Thus, we move forward, with a more serene heart and a clearer mind, ready to build relationships based on understanding, respect, and true inner peace.

# Chapter 24
# Releasing Fear

Fear arises as a natural response of the human being to situations that represent threat or uncertainty, playing a crucial role in self-preservation. However, when it exceeds the limits of balance and transforms into a persistent and disproportionate feeling, it can limit choices, block opportunities, and prevent personal growth. This emotion, when not understood, settles in as an invisible barrier that restricts the potential for fulfillment and wholeness. Recognizing fear as a reflection of past experiences and ingrained beliefs allows us to see it from a new perspective, not as an insurmountable obstacle, but as a chance for inner transformation.

Delving into the origin of fear is fundamental to dissolving its roots. Often, it manifests itself in subtle ways, masquerading as insecurity, procrastination, or self-sabotage. This emotion may have been fueled by old memories, unresolved traumas, or external influences that have consolidated patterns of limitation. By bringing these hidden layers to light, it becomes possible to question the veracity of these perceptions and begin a process of emotional healing. This internal movement of investigation allows us to reframe fear, embracing it with understanding and directing its energy towards personal empowerment.

Transforming fear into courage requires a willingness to face discomfort and break with automatic cycles of avoidance. This process involves developing self-confidence, recognizing one's own ability to overcome challenges and build new paths. Each small action taken towards facing fear reinforces inner confidence and opens space for new possibilities. Thus, the emotion that once paralyzed becomes an impulse for self-development, freeing the mind and heart to live authentically and fully.

Fear, in its essence, is an emotion deeply rooted in human nature, designed to protect and preserve life. It acts as a warning sign in the face of situations that represent danger or uncertainty, arousing attention and caution. However, when this defense mechanism intensifies disproportionately, it ceases to fulfill its protective role and begins to limit choices, block opportunities, and restrict personal growth. In these moments, fear transforms into an invisible prison, fueled by past experiences, unresolved traumas, and limiting beliefs that silently guide our decisions and behaviors.

Recognizing fear not as an enemy, but as a manifestation of internal aspects that need to be understood and healed, is the first step towards liberation. Often, it disguises itself as insecurity, procrastination, or self-sabotage, masking its deeper roots. Looking at this emotion with honesty and curiosity allows us to unravel the hidden layers that sustain fear, questioning the veracity of these perceptions and opening space for emotional healing. This internal movement is essential to reframe fear, embracing it with understanding and transforming its paralyzing energy into vital force for growth.

Transforming fear into courage requires a willingness to face discomfort and break with automatic cycles of avoidance. This process begins with self-awareness, which allows us to observe the situations that trigger fear, identify the physical sensations that accompany it, and recognize the thoughts that feed this emotion. This careful analysis reveals emotional patterns that were often formed by past experiences, but continue to influence the present. By bringing these connections to light, a process of deconstructing these beliefs begins, allowing them to be replaced by more positive and empowering perceptions.

The practice of Ho'oponopono emerges as a powerful tool on this path of liberation. Its four phrases—"I'm sorry. Please forgive me. I love you. I'm grateful."—are simple, but profoundly transformative. By directing them to the situations that trigger fear, to the people involved, or to oneself, a cleansing of the memories and beliefs that feed this emotion begins. This act of emotional purification does not seek to erase fear, but to understand it and dissolve the bonds that keep it active. With each repetition of these words, the weight of fear softens, giving way to the lightness of acceptance and courage.

Visualizing oneself facing one's fears with confidence and determination also strengthens this process. The mind has the power to shape reality, and by creating mental images of overcoming, the subconscious begins to accept the possibility of change. Imagining yourself going through challenges, achieving goals, and living with freedom reprograms the mind to act more confidently. This continuous exercise reinforces self-confidence, making facing challenging situations more natural and less frightening.

Positive affirmations are another powerful resource for dissolving fear. Phrases like "I am courageous and resilient," "I trust in my ability to overcome challenges," or "I deserve to live with freedom and joy" function as mantras that reprogram the subconscious. Repeating them daily strengthens the mind and weakens limiting beliefs, creating a new internal foundation of security and confidence. These affirmations, when aligned with concrete actions, accelerate the transformation process.

However, true overcoming of fear requires action. It is not enough to understand or visualize courage; it is necessary to put it into practice. This can start with small steps: speaking in public for a few minutes, facing a difficult conversation, trying something new. Each small victory over fear reinforces self-confidence and expands the perception that it is possible to go beyond self-imposed limitations. This positive cycle of confrontation and conquest gradually weakens fear until it loses its power to paralyze.

Compassion plays a crucial role in this process. Having compassion for yourself is understanding that feeling fear is not a sign of weakness, but a natural part of the human journey. It is allowing yourself to make mistakes, step back when necessary, and move forward when possible, without judgment or excessive demands. This kindness to oneself makes the journey lighter, as it recognizes that every step taken, however small, is a demonstration of courage. Extending this compassion to others also dissolves resentment and broadens the understanding that everyone faces their own fears.

Forgiving yourself for the times when fear prevented you from moving forward is also essential. Forgiveness releases the weight of guilt and creates space for new attempts. It allows the past to be seen as learning, not as a prison. Forgiving also those who, in some way, contributed to the formation of fears and insecurities is an act of liberation, as it takes away from them the power over our emotions. This movement of forgiveness opens the way to healing and the flourishing of a lighter and more authentic life.

With time and constant practice, fear ceases to be an obstacle and becomes a silent guide, pointing to areas that need attention and growth. It comes to be seen as a sign of where there is room for evolution, not as an insurmountable barrier. This understanding completely transforms the relationship with fear, allowing it to be embraced and integrated, rather than fought or avoided. Thus, the energy previously consumed by avoidance is redirected towards self-development and personal expansion.

This journey of liberation does not mean the absence of challenges, but the construction of a new stance in the face of them. The practice of Ho'oponopono, associated with the cultivation of self-confidence, strengthens emotional resilience, broadening the understanding that each obstacle contains an opportunity for growth. Life begins to be lived with more lightness, authenticity, and purpose, for fear, once oppressive, is now seen as an opportunity for evolution and strengthening.

With a lighter heart and an open mind, it becomes possible to embrace the unknown with courage and curiosity. True freedom lies not in the absence of risks, but in the confidence that each step is guided by inner wisdom. From this perspective, fear dissolves in the face of the clarity of those who choose to live fully, allowing each experience, positive or challenging, to contribute to the construction of a rich, meaningful, and authentic journey. Thus, freeing oneself from fear is, above all, allowing oneself to live fully, expanding one's horizons and embracing all the possibilities that life has to offer.

By treading this path of self-knowledge and healing, one realizes that fear ceases to be a burden and transforms into a silent guide, pointing to areas that need attention and care. Each confrontation, however small, represents a victory over internal limitations and reinforces the connection with one's own essence. Thus, the liberation process becomes continuous, allowing new possibilities to flourish where before there was only stagnation and insecurity.

This movement of inner expansion does not mean the absence of challenges, but a new posture in the face of them. The constant practice of Ho'oponopono, combined with the cultivation of self-confidence, strengthens emotional resilience and broadens the understanding that each obstacle carries within itself an opportunity for growth. Life begins to be lived with more lightness, authenticity, and purpose, for fear, once oppressive, now serves as a reminder of the infinite capacity for adaptation and overcoming.

With a lighter heart and an open mind, it becomes possible to embrace the unknown with courage and curiosity. The freedom gained does not lie in the absence of risks, but in the unwavering confidence that each step is guided by inner wisdom. Thus, fear dissolves in the face of the clarity of those who choose to live fully, allowing each experience to contribute to the construction of a rich, meaningful, and authentic journey.

# Chapter 25
# Anxiety: Calming the Mind

The restless mind, dominated by racing thoughts and constant worries, reflects a state of continuous alertness that wears down emotional and physical balance. Anxiety arises in this scenario as an automatic response, often disproportionate, that consumes vital energy and prevents the full experience of the present. This incessant flow of anticipatory thoughts creates a cycle of tension that weakens the ability to deal with daily challenges. Recognizing anxiety as a manifestation of memories and limiting beliefs allows one to begin a process of inner transformation, in which it is possible to slow down the mind and restore tranquility.

A deep understanding of anxiety reveals that it is not an insurmountable obstacle, but a sign that unresolved emotional aspects are asking for attention. From this understanding, it becomes feasible to access the roots of this restlessness, identifying thought patterns and repressed emotions that sustain this mental state. This conscious approach opens space to question the origin of these worries, gradually dissolving the impact they have on the mind and body. Thus, it is possible to break the cycle of anxiety and rebuild a foundation of serenity and confidence.

By adopting practices that favor connection with the present moment, the mind naturally slows down, allowing the body to relax and emotions to stabilize. Deep breathing techniques, guided meditation, and positive affirmations are effective resources for bringing the mind back into balance. These practices, when performed regularly, strengthen the ability to observe thoughts without getting caught up in them, promoting a lasting sense of calm and mental clarity. This continuous process of self-care not only relieves anxiety, but also expands self-awareness, creating an internal environment conducive to well-being and harmony.

Anxiety manifests as a constant stream of racing thoughts and intense emotions, creating a state of continuous alertness that wears down both mind and body. This mental whirlwind, fueled by worries about the future or memories of the past, directly interferes with the ability to live the present moment fully. The restless mind, filled with uncertainties and fears, triggers physical and emotional reactions that affect overall well-being. Muscle tension, insomnia, irritability, and difficulty concentrating are just some of the signs that inner balance has been compromised. In this scenario, recognizing anxiety as a reflection of ingrained memories and beliefs becomes the first step in transforming it and restoring inner tranquility.

Understanding that anxiety is a learned response to situations of insecurity allows us to investigate its deeper causes. Often, this emotional state is sustained by unprocessed past experiences, silent traumas, or patterns of negative thinking that repeat themselves over time.

Awareness of these roots makes it possible to question the veracity of the beliefs that fuel fear and worry, opening space to reframe them. It is in this process of investigation and understanding that Ho'oponopono presents itself as an effective practice to dissolve the layers of anxiety, promoting a state of peace and balance.

Ho'oponopono, with its four simple phrases—"I'm sorry. Please forgive me. I love you. I'm grateful."—acts as a powerful tool to cleanse the memories that sustain anxiety. By repeating these words with intention, it is possible to release emotional patterns that keep the mind trapped in cycles of worry. This purification process does not seek to deny anxiety, but to embrace it with compassion, allowing its energy to be gently dissolved. Each repetition of these phrases deepens the connection with the present moment, reducing the influence of disturbing thoughts and creating space for serenity.

Observing anxiety with attention and without judgment is another fundamental step. Identifying the triggers that awaken it, the associated physical sensations, and the thoughts that reinforce it broaden the understanding of how it operates. This attentive and compassionate look helps to interrupt the automatic cycle of reaction, making it possible to respond to situations in a more balanced way. This awareness is liberating, as it gives back the power of choice over how to deal with emotions, taking away the idea that anxiety has absolute control over life.

The practice of mindful breathing is an accessible and effective tool to calm the anxious mind. Breathing slowly and deeply activates the parasympathetic nervous system, responsible for relaxing the body. This simple act of paying attention to the breath slows the heartbeat, reduces muscle tension, and creates an immediate sense of calm. Regular mindful breathing practices help interrupt the flow of anxious thoughts, bringing the mind back to the present and promoting emotional balance.

Combined with breathing, meditation is a practice that silences the restless mind and restores inner clarity. Dedicating a few minutes each day to guided meditation or observing your own breathing creates a space of stillness where anxiety finds no ground to expand. Meditation teaches you to observe thoughts without identifying with them, allowing them to come and go without causing suffering. This healthy detachment from the restless mind promotes emotional stability and expands the ability to face challenges with more serenity.

Positive visualizations are also effective resources to combat anxiety. Imagining yourself in peaceful environments, surrounded by nature or enveloped by soft light, provides immediate relief and conditions the mind to seek states of calm. Visualizing challenging situations being faced with confidence and balance reinforces the idea that it is possible to act safely even in the face of discomfort. These mental images function as rehearsals for the brain, training it to respond more calmly to adversity.

Positive affirmations complement this transformation process. Repeating phrases such as "I am calm and confident," "I release anxiety and embrace peace," or "I trust the flow of life" reprograms the subconscious, weakening negative thought patterns. This daily habit strengthens self-confidence and creates a new internal foundation of security, gradually dissolving the dominance of anxiety.

However, it is conscious action that consolidates the overcoming of anxiety. Small practical steps, such as organizing daily tasks, setting priorities, or gradually facing situations that cause discomfort, are fundamental to building confidence. Each small victory reinforces the perception that anxiety does not have absolute power and that it is possible to live with more lightness. The combination of self-awareness, relaxation practices, and concrete action generates a positive cycle of growth and emotional strengthening.

Self-compassion is essential in this process. It is important to understand that feeling anxious is not a sign of weakness, but a natural response to challenges. Treating yourself with kindness, respecting your own limits, and acknowledging the efforts made to overcome this emotional state make the journey lighter. Self-compassion opens space for welcoming emotions, reducing self-criticism, and encouraging the search for balance in a more loving and patient way.

Over time, the constant practice of Ho'oponopono and other self-care techniques transforms the relationship with anxiety. What was once seen as an obstacle becomes recognized as a sign that something needs to be taken care of. This more compassionate and attentive look allows one to deal with anxiety in a more balanced way, recognizing that each thought and emotion can be understood, embraced, and transformed.

This journey of self-knowledge and healing does not seek to completely eliminate anxiety, but to reduce its impact and strengthen the ability to face it with serenity. With each practice, the mind becomes clearer and more focused, and the body responds with relaxation and balance. Anxiety ceases to dominate actions and becomes just a fleeting emotion that arises and dissipates without causing prolonged suffering.

Thus, cultivating inner peace through Ho'oponopono and self-care practices is a daily commitment to one's own well-being. This path of love and acceptance allows one to go through life's challenges with more confidence and lightness. By taking care of the mind and heart, one opens space to live with more presence, gratitude, and serenity, building a fuller life, balanced and aligned with the true purpose of being.

Integrating Ho'oponopono as a constant practice allows the journey of self-knowledge to become deeper and more meaningful. Each repetition of the simple phrases carries the intention of healing and release, dissolving layers of repressed emotions and limiting thoughts. This gradual process strengthens emotional resilience, offering a new perspective on daily challenges. Anxiety, once seen as an obstacle, is transformed into a sign that there is room for growth and inner evolution.

Over time, the conscious practice of these techniques creates a solid foundation of self-control and serenity. Small daily changes, such as moments of silence, deep breaths, or simple repetitions of mantras, accumulate into a more balanced state of being. This inner harmony is reflected in attitudes, decisions, and relationships, making life lighter and more meaningful. The mind, once scattered and anxious, begins to operate with more clarity and purpose.

Thus, cultivating inner peace through Ho'oponopono and self-care practices is a continuous path of love and acceptance. This commitment to oneself allows one to go through life's uncertainties with more confidence, recognizing that each thought and emotion can be transformed. By taking care of the mind and heart, one opens space to live with more presence, gratitude, and serenity, creating a fuller existence aligned with true balance.

# Chapter 26
# Depression, Self-Healing and Hope

The experience of depression represents a challenging journey marked by feelings of emptiness, deep sadness, and disconnection from one's own essence. This emotional state does not arise suddenly, but as a result of an accumulation of painful experiences, limiting beliefs, and unresolved emotional patterns. The mind becomes dominated by negative and self-deprecating thoughts, while the body responds with constant fatigue and loss of vitality. In this scenario, the perception of oneself and the world becomes distorted, obscuring the possibility of change and renewal. However, understanding depression as a sign of internal imbalance and not as a personal weakness is the first step in taking a path of healing and reconnection with life.

Self-healing begins with acceptance of one's own suffering and with the willingness to look inward, recognizing the emotional wounds that need to be cared for. This process involves embracing one's own vulnerability with kindness, allowing oneself to feel without judgment. Self-compassion becomes an essential foundation on this journey, as it strengthens the ability to care for oneself with patience and love. Each small step taken towards well-being is a victory, however discreet, and should be recognized as part of a continuous movement of transformation. From this perspective, it is possible to gradually free oneself from emotional bonds and open space for the renewal of hope.

By cultivating practices that favor emotional balance and reconnection with one's essence, the inner light begins to expand, slowly dissipating the darkness. The search for small sources of gratitude in everyday life, the strengthening of emotional bonds, and care for the body and mind contribute significantly to restoring well-being. The journey to overcome depression takes time, patience, and persistence, but it also reveals the inner strength capable of leading to renewal. In this process, hope is reborn, bringing with it the possibility of a lighter, more authentic life full of meaning.

Depression, often described as a shadow that settles in the soul, manifests itself in varied and subtle ways, affecting both body and mind. It is not just a passing feeling of sadness, but deepens into a loss of interest in previously enjoyed activities, accompanied by a persistent fatigue that seems to exhaust any will to act. Concentration becomes a daily challenge, while appetite and sleep become dysregulated, increasing the feeling of disconnection from one's own body. Negative thoughts arise frequently, feeding feelings of guilt and worthlessness that further isolate the individual from their social relationships. This silent cycle affects not only those who experience it, but also the people around them, who often do not understand the depth of this invisible suffering.

Within this bleak scenario, the ancestral practice of Ho'oponopono emerges as a proposal for reconciliation and inner healing. More than a simple ritual, this Hawaiian teaching invites reflection that depression should not be seen as a weakness or a character flaw. On the contrary, it can be understood as an urgent request for healing, a call to turn inward and identify memories and beliefs that imprison the mind in darkness. By adopting this perspective, the practice of Ho'oponopono becomes a tool of liberation, offering the possibility of breaking the cycle of emotional pain and rediscovering the light of hope that, although weakened, never completely fades away.

However, it is important to understand that Ho'oponopono does not replace conventional medical treatment. Caring for mental health requires the active participation of specialized professionals, such as psychologists, psychiatrists, and therapists, who can offer proper diagnosis and effective therapeutic interventions. Still, Ho'oponopono can act as a valuable complement in this process, aiding in self-healing and alleviating symptoms, while strengthening the connection with one's essence and reviving the joy of living.

The practice of Ho'oponopono is structured on pillars that favor self-healing and overcoming depression. The first of these is responsibility. Taking responsibility for one's own healing does not mean carrying the weight of guilt, but recognizing that, even in the midst of suffering, there is a personal power of transformation. It is an invitation to realize that, despite adversity, there is the possibility of shaping one's own reality and actively seeking happiness. This step is essential, as it awakens the awareness that small changes can trigger major transformations.

Another fundamental aspect is self-compassion. Cultivating an attitude of affection and understanding towards oneself allows one to recognize pain without judgment and offer oneself the necessary care for recovery. Self-compassion is a foundation that sustains the healing journey, helping to dissolve self-deprecating thoughts and allowing the construction of a more welcoming and safe inner space. This process does not require grand gestures, but begins with simple attitudes, such as respecting one's own limits and validating each achievement, however small.

Memory cleansing is one of the central points of Ho'oponopono. Through the four phrases—"I'm sorry. Please forgive me. I love you. I'm grateful."—an inner dialogue of acceptance and release begins. These words, when directed at negative thoughts and feelings of sadness, guilt, and worthlessness, have the power to soften the weight of past experiences. The conscious repetition of these phrases acts as a key that unlocks doors locked by pain, allowing repressed emotions to be embraced and transformed. It is a delicate and gradual process, but deeply effective in dissolving emotional patterns that feed depression.

Gratitude, often neglected during periods of suffering, proves to be a powerful tool for reconnecting with life. Finding small reasons to be grateful—whether for a ray of sunshine warming the skin, the aroma of coffee in the morning, or the comfort of a hug—rescues the ability to perceive the beauty that still exists around us. The daily practice of gratitude does not eliminate pain immediately, but it broadens the perception that, even in the midst of darkness, there are sparks of light that can be cultivated. This shift in focus not only strengthens emotional resilience but also nourishes the hope of lighter days.

Recognizing one's own divine essence is another essential step in the practice of Ho'oponopono. Regardless of the suffering faced, there is an inner light that remains intact, waiting to be rediscovered. Connecting with this divine spark does not require specific beliefs, but rather the acceptance that there is something greater sustaining one's own existence. By allowing this inner light to guide the healing process, a solid foundation is created to face challenges with more courage and serenity.

Celebrating small steps is an attitude that strengthens the healing journey. Each step forward, however small it may seem, represents a significant victory. Getting out of bed on a difficult day, going for a walk for a few minutes, or simply breathing consciously are gestures that demonstrate inner strength. Recognizing these progresses with kindness and respect reinforces the perception that recovery is not linear, but made of moments of progress and setbacks, all equally important.

Seeking support is also a vital component on this path. Loneliness aggravates pain, but sharing experiences can bring relief and understanding. Being surrounded by people who offer genuine love or participating in support groups provides a safe space to express emotions and receive support. This network of acceptance does not eliminate pain, but softens the weight it imposes, creating an environment conducive to the flourishing of hope.

Even when depression makes it seem like happiness is unattainable and darkness is permanent, Ho'oponopono reminds us that the light never completely disappears. It may be hidden, weakened, but it is still there, waiting to be accessed. The healing process does not happen abruptly; it happens slowly, step by step, respecting the rhythm of each person. Allowing oneself to live this process, with constancy and gentleness, is fundamental to opening space for renewal.

Thus, the integration of practices such as Ho'oponopono with medical treatments and therapeutic support builds a solid foundation for overcoming depression. This path allows new perceptions to flourish, bringing clarity where there was once confusion and awakening the ability to see possibilities where there were only obstacles. Reconnecting with one's essence also involves appreciating the small joys of everyday life—observing the sky, feeling the breeze, listening to welcoming music. It is these simple moments that rescue the feeling of belonging to life.

Over time, pain gives way to a deeper understanding of oneself and one's own journey. Depression, once perceived as an unbearable burden, is transformed into an opportunity for growth and reconnection. The inner light, nurtured by self-compassion, sincere support, and commitment to one's own healing, becomes a gentle guide on the way back to life. In this continuous and delicate process, hope is reborn—not as a distant ideal, but as a real presence, capable of sustaining a lighter, more authentic, and purposeful life.

Allowing oneself to experience the healing process is recognizing that each stage, however subtle, carries a profound meaning. The path out of darkness does not require haste, but rather constancy and gentleness with one's own limits. By integrating practices such as Ho'oponopono with medical treatments and therapeutic support, a solid foundation for overcoming is built. This combination of care opens space for new perceptions to emerge, awakening the ability to see possibilities where there were once only obstacles.

Reconnecting with one's essence also involves recognizing the small daily joys. Watching the sunrise, feeling the breeze on your face, or simply listening to music that brings comfort are simple but powerful gestures that rescue the feeling of belonging to life. Each moment of genuine presence contributes to dissolving the feeling of isolation and strengthens hope. Thus, self-care ceases to be an isolated effort and is transformed into a continuous flow of self-love and renewal.

Over time, pain gives way to a deeper understanding of oneself and one's own journey. Depression, once an unbearable weight, is transformed into an opportunity for growth and reconnection. The inner light, nurtured by self-compassion, sincere support, and commitment to one's own healing, gently guides the way back to life. And it is in this process, step by step, that hope is reborn—not as something distant, but as a real and constant presence, capable of sustaining a lighter, more authentic, and purposeful life.

# Chapter 27
# Consolation in the Pain of Loss

The pain of loss is an experience that deeply touches the soul, awakening intense feelings of sadness, emptiness, and longing. When a loved one departs, their absence becomes overwhelmingly present, bringing to the surface the vulnerability and fragility of existence. This moment of farewell is not limited to the end of a shared life but involves the re-signification of bonds and adaptation to a new reality. Navigating grief requires delicacy and understanding, as each emotion that emerges carries with it the expression of love and lived connection. Allowing oneself to feel this pain, without resistance or judgment, is an essential step to begin the healing process.

The path to finding consolation in pain involves embracing memories with affection and respect, recognizing that the bond with the departed remains alive in memory and heart. Longing, although painful, can be transformed into a bridge connecting the past to the continuity of life. Cultivating moments of reflection and gratitude for shared moments strengthens the feeling of presence, even in the face of physical absence. This process does not seek to erase the pain but to soften it with the recognition that the love experienced transcends time and space, offering comfort and serenity.

By embracing one's pain with compassion, the possibility arises of transforming suffering into a profound learning experience about life, love, and impermanence. This inner movement paves the way to honor the memory of the departed with gestures of affection and celebration, keeping alive the essence of the relationship built. From this perspective, the pain of loss can be gently transformed into strength, allowing one to move forward with courage, hope, and the certainty that each life story remains eternally etched in the heart.

Grief is a silent and profound journey, a crossing that requires courage and delicacy. Each person experiences this pain in a unique way, with their own nuances of feelings and thoughts. There are no rules or deadlines for overcoming the loss of a loved one. Sadness, longing, anger, guilt, and even confusion emerge as unpredictable waves, bringing to the surface the intensity of the bond that existed. Allowing oneself to feel these emotions without judgment is a gesture of respect for one's pain and a way to honor the love that was shared. Grief, after all, is not weakness, but a legitimate expression of affection and connection with the departed.

Within this challenging journey, the practice of Ho'oponopono emerges as a beacon of serenity, illuminating the path of emotional healing. This Hawaiian philosophy teaches that grief is an opportunity for reconciliation and inner healing. It is not about forgetting or minimizing pain but accepting loss as an inevitable part of the cycle of life. This acceptance does not imply moving away from the love one feels, but recognizing that although the physical presence has departed, the bond remains alive in memories and in the heart. It is in this intimate space that one can find comfort and begin the delicate process of transforming pain into serenity.

Honoring the memory of the departed becomes a way to keep the connection alive. Keeping photos, remembering stories, and preserving objects that refer to special moments are subtle ways to celebrate life and the legacy left behind. Small rituals, such as lighting a candle in tribute or dedicating a prayer, help transform longing into a serene presence. These gestures do not erase the absence, but they re-signify the void, allowing love to continue to flourish silently and constantly.

Expressing emotions is essential in this process. Keeping pain silent can intensify suffering, while releasing feelings offers space for healing. Allowing oneself to cry, talk to friends or family, write about pain in a diary, or express it through art are ways to give voice to the emotions that echo in the heart. Ho'oponopono, with its four phrases — "I'm sorry. Please forgive me. I love you. I'm grateful." — acts as an emotional cleansing practice. These words, repeated with sincerity, can be directed to the loved one who has passed, to oneself, and to the situations that generated pain. This practice does not seek to erase the memory but to alleviate the weight of unresolved emotions.

Forgiveness is another important pillar on the grief journey. Often, loss awakens feelings of guilt or regret for unspoken words or unrealized gestures. Forgiving yourself for what was left unsaid or undone, as well as forgiving the loved one for any disagreements, is an act of liberation. Forgiveness does not diminish the pain of absence, but it softens the edges of suffering, opening the way to inner peace. Freeing oneself from these emotional burdens allows one to move forward with more lightness and serenity.

Gratitude, even in the midst of pain, has transformative power. Giving thanks for the moments lived, for the shared laughter, and for the lessons learned strengthens the heart. Recognizing the beauty of what was lived does not nullify the sadness of loss but creates a bridge between pain and hope. This feeling of gratitude softens the rigidity of grief and rescues the perception that, despite the absence, love remains as an eternal bond. Ho'oponopono reminds us that by cultivating gratitude, we strengthen the connection with love that transcends farewell.

Spiritual connection also plays a fundamental role in this healing process. Each person finds comfort in different forms of spirituality, whether through faith, meditation, or practices that nourish the soul. Connecting with one's own divine essence or with personal beliefs offers support in moments of fragility. This intimate contact with the sacred can bring answers, comfort, and, above all, the feeling that the journey of life does not end with death. Spirituality becomes a source of comfort, reminding us that existence is continuous and that love knows no bounds.

Celebrating the life of the departed is a way to honor their memory with joy and respect. Planting a tree in tribute, dedicating moments of reflection, or even helping someone on behalf of the loved one are ways to keep love in motion. These simple but profound gestures transform the pain of absence into a legacy of affection and meaning. They show that although the farewell was inevitable, the impact of the departed continues to reverberate in the world through concrete and loving actions.

It is crucial to remember that grief need not be faced alone. Seeking support from friends, family, or support groups offers a safe space to share pain and find understanding. Specialized professionals, such as psychologists and therapists, can help in understanding and welcoming emotions, offering tools to deal with suffering. The attentive listening and support of those who understand the depth of this pain are essential to go through grief with more resilience.

Ho'oponopono invites the reflection that grief, however painful, is not an end, but a transition. The pain of loss never completely disappears, but with time, it transforms. It can soften, becoming a quiet longing that accompanies but does not paralyze. The love lived remains, shaping how each one chooses to move forward. This continuous healing process allows one to find new meaning for absence, where memory becomes inspiration and love is reflected in every choice to live with more presence and gratitude.

Allowing oneself to experience grief authentically is a way of honoring not only the departed but also one's own life. Each tear, each silence, and each memory is part of a natural cycle of healing that happens at the pace of each heart. There is no hurry to silence the pain because it is a reflection of the deep love that existed. By embracing this vulnerability, space is opened for longing to transform into a gentle presence that inspires new paths.

Thus, the pain of loss can, over time, be softened by gestures of love and understanding. Planting a tree in tribute, writing letters, or simply reserving moments of silence are ways to keep the connection alive with the departed. These rituals do not nullify the absence, but they help to re-signify it, allowing life to continue with more lightness. Ho'oponopono, in this context, serves as a constant reminder that love does not dissolve with farewell; it transforms and continues to inhabit our hearts.

Finding comfort in the pain of loss is understanding that life is made of encounters and farewells, but also of bonds that time does not break. Honoring the departed is also honoring oneself, allowing oneself to live with authenticity, lightness, and gratitude. And, in this process, hope is reborn as a soft light, guiding the heart and giving meaning to the new stages that unfold along the way. The love lived remains, eternal and silent, like a beacon that illuminates and guides, even on the darkest nights.

Allowing oneself to experience grief authentically is an act of self-love and respect for the history shared with the departed. Each tear shed, each profound silence, and each memory rescued are part of a healing process that happens in one's own time. There is no hurry to silence the pain because it carries the depth of the bond and the importance of who was lost. By accepting this vulnerability, space is opened for longing to gradually transform into a serene presence that accompanies and inspires new paths.

Over time, small gestures can become powerful rituals of reconnection with the memory of the departed. Planting a tree, writing letters, or simply dedicating moments of reflection are subtle but meaningful ways to keep love and gratitude alive. These practices do not nullify the absence, but they help to re-signify it, allowing life to move forward with more lightness. Ho'oponopono, in this context, acts as a constant reminder that love does not dissolve with farewell, but transforms and continues to flourish within us.

Thus, finding comfort in the pain of loss is understanding that the cycle of life involves encounters and farewells, but also eternal connections that are not broken over time. Honoring the departed is also honoring one's own life, allowing oneself to live with authenticity, lightness, and gratitude. And, in this process, hope is reborn, bringing with it the certainty that the love lived remains as a soft light that guides the heart, giving meaning to the new stages that unfold along the way.

# Chapter 28
# Freeing Yourself from the Bonds of the Past

Forgiveness is revealed as a transformative force capable of dissolving the emotional barriers that keep people trapped in past pain. It is a profound act of love and compassion, which allows the release of resentment, guilt, and hurt accumulated over time. By adopting forgiveness as a conscious practice, there is a release of emotional burdens that prevent personal growth and the achievement of a lighter and fuller life. This process does not require the approval or understanding of others, but rather a personal commitment to one's own healing and evolution. Recognizing the importance of forgiveness is the first step to undoing the knots that connect us to painful experiences, allowing peace and harmony to flow freely in all aspects of life.

The decision to forgive implies courage to revisit deep feelings and look at oneself with honesty and compassion. This inner movement promotes the acceptance of human imperfections and the understanding that mistakes are part of learning. By allowing forgiveness to flow, one does not deny the pain experienced, but chooses not to feed it anymore, creating space for inner renewal. This emotional openness favors the dissolution of negative patterns and enables a new way of relating to oneself and others. Thus, forgiveness is consolidated as an essential pillar for the reconstruction of self-esteem, for emotional strengthening, and for the construction of healthier and more balanced relationships.

By integrating forgiveness as a constant practice, a profound transformation occurs in the way life's challenges are experienced. The emotional lightness achieved is reflected in more compassionate and empathetic attitudes, expanding the capacity to deal with adversity with serenity. This continuous process of self-healing reinforces the connection with one's essence and awakens a genuine feeling of gratitude for the journey traveled. Thus, by choosing the path of forgiveness, one opens the possibility of living a fuller life, full of love, understanding, and emotional freedom, where the past no longer dictates the rhythm of the present, and the future is built with more lightness and authenticity.

Freeing oneself from the bonds of the past is a profound process of transformation that requires courage, patience, and compassion. Forgiveness, in this context, emerges as an essential key to dissolving the emotional barriers that keep people trapped in hurt, resentment, and guilt accumulated throughout life. It is not about forgetting or justifying the pain experienced, but about consciously choosing to let go of the weight that prevents the natural flow of life. This intimate decision to release suffering allows inner peace and self-love to flourish, creating space for personal growth and the construction of a lighter and more authentic existence. By recognizing that forgiveness is a gesture of self-love and not of submission, the path to true emotional freedom is opened.

Forgiving involves revisiting deep wounds with honesty and kindness. This inner dive does not deny the pain felt but seeks to understand and re-signify it. It is an act of courage to look at one's own mistakes and the failures of others with the understanding that imperfection is part of the human experience. This compassionate gaze transforms pain into learning and allows one to undo the knots that imprison the heart. By allowing forgiveness to flow, we stop feeding hurt and resentment, creating space for inner renewal and a new way of relating to oneself and the world.

Ho'oponopono, a Hawaiian practice of reconciliation and healing, offers valuable tools for this liberation process. Its four phrases — "I'm sorry. Please forgive me. I love you. I'm grateful." — are more than just words; they are an invitation to cleanse painful memories and restore emotional balance. When repeated with sincere intention, these phrases act as a balm for the wounded heart, dissolving resentment and softening the weight of the past. Ho'oponopono teaches us that forgiving does not require the participation of the other, as it is an internal movement of healing that frees those who decide to move on without carrying hurt.

Self-forgiveness is perhaps the most profound challenge on this journey. Often, we are our own biggest critics, judging ourselves harshly for past choices, for unspoken words, or for actions that have brought pain to ourselves or others. Carrying this weight hinders evolution and personal flourishing. Forgiving oneself is recognizing one's own humanity, accepting limitations, and understanding that each decision was made with the emotional and mental resources available at that time. This act of inner compassion is liberating because it allows one to start over with lightness and with the wisdom acquired through lived experiences.

In relationships, forgiveness plays a fundamental role. Harboring resentment and hurt creates invisible barriers that prevent harmony and joint growth. When we forgive someone who has hurt us, we are not erasing what happened, but we are choosing not to carry the weight of that pain anymore. This gesture frees stagnant energy and opens space for reconciliation, if possible, or for inner peace, even if both paths continue in different directions. Forgiveness, in this context, does not require continuous coexistence with the one who caused pain, but offers the opportunity to move on without the burden of hurt.

By practicing forgiveness, we also develop empathy and understanding. When we recognize our own faults and forgive ourselves, we become more compassionate towards the mistakes of others. This empathy strengthens emotional bonds and promotes healthier and more authentic relationships. From this point, we build bonds based on mutual understanding and respect, making a more harmonious coexistence possible.

Freeing oneself from the past also involves emotional detachment. Often, we get stuck in situations or with people because of unmet expectations or unresolved pain. Forgiveness is the way to undo these ties that bind us to moments that have already passed. By releasing resentment, we open space for new experiences and opportunities for growth. This detachment does not mean devaluing what has been lived, but understanding that life is in constant motion and that the present deserves to be lived fully.

Ho'oponopono reinforces that although the past cannot be changed, the way we relate to it can be transformed. By choosing forgiveness, we rewrite our history from a new perspective, freeing ourselves from old pain and creating a lighter and happier path. This healing process is continuous and requires daily practice, but each step taken represents a significant advance towards inner peace.

Forgiveness also leads us to a path of love and compassion. Not only for the other, but mainly for ourselves. It is a silent and profound gift that we offer to our hearts. By releasing the bonds of pain, we open space for joy, serenity, and fullness. This conscious choice to cultivate peace, even in the face of adversity, strengthens the soul and awakens a new perspective on life.

Moving forward with a light heart is one of the greatest gifts we can offer ourselves. By freeing ourselves from the chains of the past, we create space to live the present fully and to build a more harmonious future. Forgiveness guides us on a journey of self-knowledge and unconditional love, where we learn that true strength lies in choosing peace. On this path, each experience, however painful it may have been, becomes part of a greater learning experience that leads us to a more serene and authentic existence.

Practicing forgiveness is not an isolated act, but a continuous choice. Each time we choose to forgive, we are reaffirming our commitment to emotional freedom and our evolution. This process reconnects us with our essence, making us more resilient in the face of adversity and more open to love and joy. Thus, forgiveness is consolidated as a path of deep healing, which leads us to a lighter, truer, and fuller life.

By integrating forgiveness as part of our journey, we open space for love and gratitude to flow freely. This inner movement frees and strengthens us, allowing the pain of the past to no longer dictate the rhythm of our present. Thus, we build a future full of possibilities, where each step is guided by lightness, compassion, and authenticity. In this liberation process, we find not only peace, but also the opportunity to flourish and to live with more truth and depth.

Freeing oneself from the bonds of the past is recognizing that the pain experienced does not define who we are, but can be transformed into learning and growth. Forgiveness does not erase what happened, but softens the emotional weight we carry, allowing new possibilities to flourish. By letting go of hurt and releasing resentment, we create space to rebuild our paths with more lightness and authenticity. This movement of emotional detachment does not happen immediately, but each step taken in this direction represents a significant advance towards inner freedom.

The constant practice of Ho'oponopono strengthens this liberation process, acting as a daily reminder that we can choose peace instead of pain. By repeating the phrases with sincerity, we gradually dissolve inner blockages and allow self-love to manifest itself more strongly. This emotional openness connects us with our truest essence, making us more empathetic and understanding, both with our own faults and with the limitations of others. Thus, forgiveness ceases to be just an isolated act and becomes a continuous practice of self-care and evolution.

Moving forward with a light heart is a gift we give ourselves. When we free ourselves from the chains of the past, we open the way to live fully in the present and build a more harmonious future. Forgiveness leads us on a journey of self-knowledge and unconditional love, where we learn that true strength lies in choosing peace. On this path, each experience becomes part of a greater learning experience, guiding us to a more serene, authentic, and deeply connected life with the now.

# Chapter 29
# Connecting with the Divine Essence

Connecting with the divine essence is a journey of self-discovery and deep integration with the creative force that permeates the universe. This connection transcends religious beliefs and dogmas, allowing each individual to recognize the presence of the divine in themselves and in others. It is about understanding that we are parts of a greater whole, interconnected by a subtle energy that guides life and sustains existence. By opening ourselves to this awareness, we awaken to inner wisdom, expand our perception of reality, and harmonize with the natural and spiritual laws that govern the cosmos. This integration provides emotional balance, mental clarity, and serenity in the face of challenges, fostering a life guided by love, compassion, and gratitude.

This connection with the divine essence does not require complex rituals or rigid practices; it manifests through simple but profound attitudes, such as cultivating inner silence, listening to intuition, and the constant practice of forgiveness. By accessing this state of conscious presence, we open space for inner healing and reconciliation with all parts of ourselves. This integration leads us to recognize that each experience lived, whether of pain or joy, is part of a larger process of learning and evolution. Thus, the search for this connection becomes a path of self-transformation, in which the illusion of separation dissolves and the sense of unity with all that exists is strengthened.

By aligning ourselves with this spiritual dimension, we develop the ability to live with more authenticity and purpose. We begin to understand that our actions, thoughts, and feelings reverberate in the collective, influencing not only our own lives but also the environment around us. This awareness drives us to act with responsibility, empathy, and generosity, contributing to the construction of a more harmonious world. From this connection, a deeper understanding of the meaning of existence flourishes, allowing life to be guided by the wisdom of the heart and the certainty that we are co-creators of our reality. Thus, by strengthening this bond with the divine essence, we open paths to a fuller, lighter existence in tune with the natural flow of life.

Connecting with the divine essence is a journey back to what is most authentic and true within us. This path does not require rigid beliefs or complex practices, but rather a sincere openness to recognize the presence of the sacred in all that exists. It is about realizing that we are inseparable parts of a great web of life, sustained by a universal energy that surrounds and permeates us. By aligning ourselves with this creative force, we are invited to delve into self-knowledge and understand that each experience lived, whether of pain or joy, is part of a continuous process of learning and evolution. This awakening leads us to a lighter life, where inner peace and harmony with the world around us become natural.

Spirituality, in this context, ceases to be a distant concept and becomes a daily experience. The simple act of silencing the mind and listening to one's own intuition already represents a step towards this connection. Small practices, such as moments of reflection, gestures of gratitude, or attentive observation of nature, bring us closer to this divine energy that inhabits each being. In this search, we recognize that the divine is not outside of us, but pulsates within us, guiding our actions and decisions. By allowing this presence to manifest, we begin to act with more compassion, responsibility, and love, both for ourselves and for others.

Ho'oponopono, as a spiritual practice, offers a bridge to this reconnection. Its four phrases — "I'm sorry. Please forgive me. I love you. I'm grateful." — are powerful tools for cleansing and realigning with our divine essence. Each word, when spoken sincerely, dissolves emotional and energetic blocks, opening space for inner peace. This practice teaches us that we are co-creators of our reality and that by taking responsibility for our thoughts and emotions, we can transform our lives. Ho'oponopono reminds us that by healing ourselves, we also contribute to the healing of the collective, for everything is interconnected.

Expanding consciousness is another fundamental step in this spiritual journey. Understanding that we are part of a greater whole frees us from the illusion of separation and strengthens the sense of unity. We begin to perceive that our actions reverberate beyond ourselves, influencing the environment and the people around us. This perception leads us to act with more empathy and generosity, recognizing that each choice has an impact on the balance of life. Living in harmony with spiritual laws — such as the law of love, gratitude, and cause and effect — guides us to a more conscious existence aligned with the principles that govern the universe.

This deep connection also awakens us to the purpose of life. From the moment we tune in to our essence, clarity arises about the role we play in the world. This purpose need not be grandiose or extraordinary; it reveals itself in small gestures of care, in words of affection, and in daily choices that reflect our commitment to good. Recognizing this purpose brings meaning to our existence, directing our steps with confidence and authenticity.

Inner peace, so longed for, is a natural result of this connection with the divine. By calming the mind and releasing negative thoughts, we find serenity even in the face of challenges. This tranquility does not mean the absence of problems, but the ability to face them with wisdom and balance. Ho'oponopono invites us to cultivate this peace through the repetition of its phrases, which function as a mantra of healing and alignment. This state of inner stillness is the basis for a full life, where each experience is welcomed as part of a greater path of evolution.

Integrating Ho'oponopono into spiritual practice is a simple and effective way to deepen this connection.

Meditation with the four phrases, for example, allows you to calm the mind and hear the voice of intuition. Prayer, by incorporating these words, becomes a moment of surrender and seeking divine guidance. Studying the principles of this practice and applying them in daily life broadens understanding of the responsibility we have in our own healing. In addition, serving others with love and compassion reinforces the idea that personal transformation reflects positively on the world around us.

This journey of reconnection with the divine essence also leads us to realize that each thought, word, and intention has a creative power. We are responsible for the energy we emanate and, consequently, for the environment we help to build. By choosing thoughts of love and gratitude, we nurture not only our own well-being but also the collective balance. Ho'oponopono, in this sense, acts as a constant reminder that we have the power to purify our mind and heart, promoting lightness and clarity on our journey.

By deepening this connection, we understand that true transformation begins from the inside out. The continuous practice of forgiveness and gratitude frees us from limiting patterns and opens us to new possibilities. This process makes us more empathetic and understanding, allowing us to relate in a healthier way with others and with the world. Thus, forgiveness ceases to be an isolated act and becomes a continuous path of evolution and care.

Living in tune with the divine essence is, therefore, living with purpose, love, and presence. Each step taken in this direction leads us to a lighter and fuller existence, where difficulties are faced with wisdom and moments of joy are lived with gratitude. By reconnecting with this greater force, we recognize that we are part of something much greater than ourselves and that each action, however small, contributes to the balance of life.

Thus, the connection with the divine essence is not a final destination, but a continuous journey of self-discovery and transformation. By allowing ourselves to experience this path with openness and authenticity, we are guided by a loving force that sustains and inspires us. Ho'oponopono offers us the tools to walk with lightness and truth, reminding us that we are responsible for our own healing and for the impact we leave on the world. In this state of unity and harmony, each choice becomes a reflection of the love that dwells within us, leading us to a fuller, truer life in tune with the natural flow of existence.

With the deepening of this spiritual journey, it becomes evident that each word, each thought, and each intention carries a power of creation and change. The constant practice of the phrases of Ho'oponopono — "I'm sorry. Please forgive me. I love you. I'm grateful." — functions as a reminder that we are co-authors of our own reality. This recognition invites us to act with more awareness and to cultivate states of love and gratitude, positively influencing not only our well-being but also the energy flow around us. It is in this process of inner purification that we find lightness and clarity to move forward, guided by a greater force that supports us.

Thus, integrating Ho'oponopono into daily spirituality is an invitation to live with more authenticity, purpose, and presence. By reconnecting with our divine essence, we awaken to the loving responsibility of caring for ourselves, others, and the planet. This path, marked by forgiveness and gratitude, reveals that true transformation begins from the inside out, leading us to a fuller, more harmonious existence aligned with the natural flow of life. In this state of unity, we understand that each step taken is part of a continuous journey of evolution and healing, where love is the force that sustains and guides each choice.

# Chapter 30
# Energetic Harmony

Energetic harmony is fundamental to maintaining balance between body, mind, and spirit, directly influencing quality of life and integral well-being. Each thought, emotion, and experience lived is reflected in the flow of vital energy, which runs through the body through specific centers called chakras. These energy vortices are responsible for regulating various physical, emotional, and spiritual functions, and their alignment is essential for energy to flow freely and healthily. When these centers are blocked or imbalanced, physical discomfort, emotional tension, and spiritual difficulties arise. Thus, caring for internal energy becomes an essential process to achieve a lighter, healthier, and fuller life.

The practice of Ho'oponopono integrates perfectly into this process, acting as a powerful tool to restore energy balance. Through the conscious repetition of the phrases "I'm sorry. Please forgive me. I love you. I'm grateful.", a deep cleansing of memories and negative patterns that compromise the flow of vital energy takes place. This simple but profound practice dissolves emotional blocks and limiting beliefs that directly affect the chakras, allowing each energy center to resume its natural functioning. With energy circulating freely, there is a revitalization of the physical body, expanded mental clarity, and a strengthening of the spiritual connection. This alignment promotes not only inner healing but also a continuous sense of peace, security, and purpose.

By integrating Ho'oponopono with visualization practices, meditation, and breathing techniques, the process of energy balance is further enhanced. Visualizing the chakras as vortices of light spinning harmoniously, feeling the energy flowing smoothly through the body, and allowing repressed emotions to be gently released are steps that amplify the effects of this connection. This holistic approach strengthens the integration between body and spirit, awakening intuition, creativity, and self-love. Thus, caring for energetic harmony becomes an act of deep self-care, capable of transforming the relationship with oneself and with the world, leading to a more balanced, healthy, and meaningful life.

In the yogic and tantric tradition, the chakras are considered essential portals of vital energy, distributed along the spine to the top of the head. Each of these energy centers plays a specific role in regulating physical, emotional, and spiritual functions. The balance of these chakras is indispensable for maintaining integral health and well-being, as any blockage or imbalance can result in physical discomfort, emotional instability, and spiritual disconnection. When vital energy flows freely and harmoniously through these points, the body achieves a state of deep balance, reflected in greater vitality, mental clarity, and emotional serenity.

The practice of Ho'oponopono emerges as a powerful and effective tool to promote the harmonization of these energy centers. By repeating with intention the phrases "I'm sorry. Please forgive me. I love you. I'm grateful.", a deep cleansing process of memories and emotional patterns begins, which often take root in the chakras, generating blockages and imbalances. This practice not only dissolves traumas and limiting beliefs but also restores the natural flow of vital energy. Each word carries a vibration capable of touching specific areas of being, providing emotional and energetic release that translates into integral well-being.

The process of harmonizing the chakras with Ho'oponopono can be intensified with conscious visualization practices. By visualizing each chakra as a vortex of light in continuous and harmonious movement, it is possible to perceive the divine energy flowing freely throughout the body. This light travels the energy pathways, dissolving subtle blockages and restoring harmony between body, mind, and spirit. This visualization not only strengthens the connection with one's own essence but also expands awareness of the impacts of repressed emotions and limiting thoughts on energy health.

Meditation also presents itself as a fundamental resource in this balancing process. Concentrating on each chakra, recognizing its location, color, and function, allows a deep immersion in the inner layers of being. During this meditative state, mantras and positive affirmations can be used to intensify the energy of each center, enhancing the cleansing promoted by Ho'oponopono. This practice leads to a state of stillness and presence, facilitating the release of old emotions and reconnection with inner wisdom.

Physical practices such as yoga and conscious breathing techniques, known as pranayama, are valuable complements in this harmonization process. Each yoga posture has been developed to stimulate specific points in the body, activating the chakras and promoting the free circulation of vital energy. Gentle movements and deep breaths create a continuous flow of energy, dissolving tension and unblocking areas that accumulate stress. This synergy between body and energy contributes to lasting balance, strengthening not only the physical body but also the emotional and spiritual.

The use of crystals is another powerful resource in harmonizing the chakras. Each crystal vibrates at an energy frequency that resonates with a specific chakra, helping to amplify and balance its energy. By positioning crystals on the body during meditation or carrying them with you in everyday life, a vibrational field is created that favors healing and energy stability. The interaction with these natural elements deepens the connection with the earth and with the subtle forces that govern inner balance.

Each chakra reflects fundamental aspects of human existence, and the practice of Ho'oponopono can directly affect the healing of these centers. The Root Chakra, located at the base of the spine, is linked to security, stability, and connection to the earth. When we carry memories of fear, abandonment, or insecurity, this center can become unbalanced, but Ho'oponopono offers a way to release these emotions, restoring the feeling of belonging and protection.

In the Sacral Chakra, associated with creativity, sexuality, and emotions, blockages can arise from experiences of guilt, shame, or emotional repression. The phrases of Ho'oponopono, directed at these memories, dissolve these barriers, allowing creative and emotional energy to flow with lightness. This process rescues spontaneity and freedom of emotional expression, essential for a full life.

The Solar Plexus Chakra, responsible for personal power and self-esteem, often accumulates energies of anger, frustration, and insecurity. Ho'oponopono acts on the transmutation of these emotions, strengthening self-confidence and willpower. This balance returns control over one's own choices and actions, allowing for more confident action in the world.

The Heart Chakra, the center of love and compassion, is deeply benefited by Ho'oponopono, a practice that encourages forgiveness and unconditional love. Taking care of this energy center promotes an opening to healthier and more loving relationships, creating an energy field that welcomes and understands the other without judgment.

In the Throat Chakra, related to communication and personal expression, memories of fear of speaking, lies, or secrets can restrict free expression. Repeating the phrases of Ho'oponopono softens these limitations, facilitating authentic and honest communication, where inner truth can be expressed without fear.

The Frontal Chakra, or Third Eye, linked to intuition and inner wisdom, can be obscured by limiting beliefs and confused thoughts. Ho'oponopono clarifies these distortions, expanding intuitive perception and a clear vision of reality. This unblock allows access to deep insights and guides life with wisdom and discernment.

Finally, the Crown Chakra, located at the top of the head, connects us to spirituality and universal consciousness. Memories that distance us from our divine essence can restrict this connection, but with Ho'oponopono, these blocks dissolve, allowing a full experience of unity with the whole. This deep connection brings peace, purpose, and understanding of interdependence with the universe.

By integrating Ho'oponopono with complementary practices such as visualization, meditation, yoga, pranayama, and the use of crystals, energy harmony is enhanced in a broad and profound way. This process not only restores the balance of the chakras, but promotes a continuous journey of self-knowledge and healing. Each step taken on this path strengthens the connection with the inner essence, leading to a more conscious, loving, and authentic existence. Thus, the practice of Ho'oponopono is revealed as a bridge between self-knowledge and universal harmony, awakening the true potential to live fully.

By promoting energy harmony through Ho'oponopono, a state of integral well-being is achieved that transcends the physical and deeply touches the emotional and spiritual. This continuous practice not only restores the balance of the chakras but also expands awareness of the interconnection between our thoughts, emotions, and the reality we live in. Vital energy flows more lightly, providing vitality, mental clarity, and emotional stability. This inner alignment is reflected in interpersonal relationships, daily choices, and the way we face challenges, leading to a lighter, more fluid existence connected to the purpose of life.

Furthermore, the integration of Ho'oponopono with complementary practices, such as the use of crystals, yoga, and meditation, enhances energy harmony and strengthens the bond with inner wisdom. This process of self-knowledge and continuous healing allows repressed emotions to be released gently, dissolving internal resistance and promoting a deep sense of peace. Thus, cultivating energy harmony becomes a daily commitment to self-care and spiritual evolution, allowing us to live more authentically, freely, and balanced.

This path of energy balance is, above all, a journey of love and reconciliation with all parts of our being. By clearing limiting memories and nurturing our energy centers with intention and compassion, we awaken to a new perception of ourselves and the world around us. The harmony achieved reverberates silently in every aspect of life, opening space for new possibilities and enriching experiences. Thus,

Ho'oponopono is revealed not only as a healing practice but as a bridge to a fuller existence, in perfect harmony with the energy of the universe.

# Chapter 31
# Healing with the Power of Sound

The transformative power of sound reveals itself as an essential tool for inner healing and emotional balance. Sacred sounds, such as mantras, possess vibrations capable of acting deeply on the mind and body, promoting well-being and reconnection with the divine essence. Integrating elevated sound practices with emotional cleansing methods amplifies the therapeutic effects, facilitating the release of limiting memories and dense emotions. This fusion of techniques not only calms the mind, but also strengthens the connection with creative energy, awakening the serenity and unconditional love present in each being.

By exploring the vibrations of mantras, an environment conducive to the harmonization of emotions and energy purification is created. Each sound chanted acts as a channel of energy that gently penetrates thoughts and feelings, dissolving inner blockages and restoring the natural flow of balance. The conscious repetition of these sacred words leads the mind to a state of presence and tranquility, allowing the body and spirit to align with higher frequencies of healing. Thus, the continuous practice of these sound vibrations enhances inner transformation and the release of limiting patterns.

Uniting emotional cleansing practices with the power of mantras creates a synergy that amplifies healing and spiritual growth. Sound resonance acts as a catalyst for forgiveness, reconciliation, and the manifestation of desires, unlocking paths to personal fulfillment. This harmonious process not only dissolves negative beliefs, but also expands consciousness, opening space for inner peace and a deep connection with universal wisdom. The vibration of sound, when combined with sincere intention, becomes a direct link with the divine source, providing integral healing and fullness.

Mantras, originating from Vedic and Buddhist traditions, are recognized as sacred instruments of healing, capable of profoundly influencing the mind, body, and spirit. Each syllable, word or phrase chanted carries a unique vibration, which resonates in the energy field of the practitioner, promoting balance and inner harmony. The attentive and intentional repetition of a mantra is not just a vocal exercise, but a dive into the subtlest layers of being, creating a direct connection with the divine essence and favoring the release of limiting emotional patterns.

When integrated with Ho'oponopono, this practice becomes even more potent. The four fundamental phrases of Ho'oponopono - "I'm sorry. Please forgive me. I love you. I'm grateful." - already act as powerful tools for emotional cleansing and reconciliation. When combined with the chanting of mantras, this purification deepens, as the sound vibrations function as catalysts, accelerating the healing process and facilitating the dissolution of energy blocks. The energy emanated by the mantras gently penetrates thoughts and emotions, restoring the natural flow of vital energy.

This fusion of practices creates a synergy that directly impacts emotional harmony. The sound resonance of mantras acts on the vibrational field of the body, calming the restless mind and softening emotional tensions. By repeating a mantra in conjunction with the Ho'oponopono phrases, a state of deep serenity and inner balance is cultivated. This state of peace allows repressed emotions to be gently released, promoting a feeling of relief and lightness. The mind slows down, the heart expands and the spirit opens to new possibilities for healing and transformation.

More than just relaxation, the combination of mantras and Ho'oponopono facilitates the reunion with the divine essence. Mantras, by their sacred nature, establish a direct bridge with the creative source of the universe. When chanted with devotion and sincere intention, they dissolve the barriers that separate us from unconditional love and fullness. Regular practice leads to an experience of unity with the whole, awakening the awareness that we are part of something greater and infinite. This perception expands compassion, strengthens empathy and inspires a more authentic life aligned with spiritual principles.

In addition to promoting healing and spiritual reconnection, mantras are also powerful tools for manifesting desires. Each sound chanted creates a specific frequency that resonates with the energy of what you want to attract. By integrating this practice with Ho'oponopono, you clear the limiting beliefs that prevent the realization of dreams and goals. The mind aligns with the vibration of abundance, allowing paths to open for the realization of personal purposes. This combination of energy cleansing and conscious manifestation strengthens self-confidence and drives personal growth.

Several mantras can be incorporated into Ho'oponopono, each with a specific vibration and purpose. The mantra "Om Gam Ganapataye Namaha", for example, is traditionally used to remove obstacles and attract prosperity. Its constant intonation dissolves internal and external barriers, creating space for new opportunities. The mantra "Om Shanti Shanti Shanti" invokes inner peace and harmony, being ideal for moments of anxiety or emotional imbalance, promoting a state of deep serenity and tranquility.

Another powerful mantra is "Om Mani Padme Hum", known for its connection to compassion and purification. This sacred sound acts directly on the heart, awakening feelings of unconditional love and understanding. For those seeking transformation and release from old patterns, the mantra "Om Namah Shivaya" is a valuable choice, as it leads the mind and spirit on paths of renewal and self-transcendence. "Om Tare Tuttare Ture Soha" is especially effective in overcoming fears and difficulties, providing courage and resilience in the face of life's challenges.

The application of mantras in Ho'oponopono can be done in several ways. Vocal or mental repetition is one of the most traditional forms, and it is important to chant the mantra with full attention and clear intention. This simple but powerful practice creates a continuous flow of energy that cleanses and harmonizes the energy field. Another approach is to use the mantra as the main focus during meditation, allowing its vibration to permeate the entire being, bringing calm and mental clarity.

Visualization is also an effective complementary technique. By imagining the mantra as a vibrant light that surrounds and penetrates the body, it is possible to enhance the cleansing of negative memories and the harmonization of internal energies. This light can be visualized dissolving blockages and filling the chakras with renewed energy. In addition, trusting your intuition to choose the right mantra for each situation is essential. Inner wisdom always guides you to the sound that most resonates with the needs of the moment, making the practice even more personalized and effective.

With the constant integration of these practices, the mind becomes more receptive and the heart more open, allowing transformative experiences to flow naturally. The journey of self-transformation becomes lighter and more fluid, as the harmony between sound and intention gently guides the dissolution of internal resistance. The vibration of mantras, combined with the compassion and forgiveness promoted by Ho'oponopono, creates a bridge that connects the individual to the natural flow of life, allowing abundance, balance and inner peace to fully manifest.

Thus, the power of sound reveals itself as an essential instrument for integral healing. By allowing these vibrations to echo in the depths of being, each individual reconnects with their true essence and with universal wisdom. This reunion not only promotes the release of old pains, but also paves the way for a fuller existence, led by serenity, love and harmony with the whole. The continuous practice of this combination transforms not only the energy field, but also the way each person relates to the world, awakening a higher consciousness and a more authentic and meaningful life.

By integrating mantras with the practice of Ho'oponopono, emotional and spiritual healing deepens organically, allowing each sound to reverberate in the subtlest layers of being. This combination creates a powerful vibrational field that dissolves accumulated tensions, expands mental clarity and strengthens intuition. The energy generated by this union enhances not only inner purification, but also facilitates reconciliation with forgotten or repressed aspects of one's own history, promoting a state of genuine and continuous peace.

With the constant use of these practices, the mind becomes more receptive and the heart more open, creating space for new experiences and perceptions. The path of self-transformation becomes lighter, as the harmony between sound and intention gently guides the dissolution of internal resistance. The vibration of mantras, combined with the compassion and forgiveness promoted by Ho'oponopono, acts as a bridge that connects the individual to the natural flow of life, allowing abundance and balance to manifest fluidly.

Thus, the power of sound, when cultivated with presence and purpose, reveals itself as an essential tool for integral healing. By allowing these vibrations to echo within, each being reconnects with their true essence and with universal wisdom. This reunion with oneself not only promotes the release of old pains, but also paves the way for a fuller existence, guided by serenity, love and harmony with the whole.

# Chapter 32
# Law of Attraction

The connection between Ho'oponopono and the Law of Attraction reveals a powerful integration of practices that enhance the conscious creation of reality. Both share the premise that thoughts, emotions and beliefs shape the experiences lived, with individual responsibility being the central point of this process. By uniting the cleansing of memories from Ho'oponopono with the positive vibration proposed by the Law of Attraction, it is possible to unblock limiting patterns and allow abundance, love and fulfillment to flow naturally. This combination strengthens the ability to manifest desires, making the co-creation process more conscious and aligned with the inner essence.

This integration is not limited to eliminating negative beliefs, but also involves cultivating elevated emotions that resonate with what you want to attract. Feelings such as gratitude, joy and love become powerful emitters of energy, aligning the individual with frequencies that attract positive experiences. Ho'oponopono, by promoting the purification of memories and emotional traumas, facilitates this vibrational alignment, allowing the Law of Attraction to act more effectively. Thus, clear thoughts and positive emotions begin to operate as catalysts for the achievement of goals and dreams.

Furthermore, the conscious practice of visualizing goals clearly and acting with confidence amplifies the power of manifestation. The combination of these practices encourages an active stance towards life, where confidence and determination replace fear and insecurity. This balance between thought, emotion and action creates an energy field conducive to transforming desires into reality. By taking responsibility for their journey and aligning with universal wisdom, each person can access a state of fullness and fulfillment, co-creating a life rich in meaning, purpose and happiness.

The Law of Attraction and Ho'oponopono converge on an essential point: individual responsibility in creating one's own reality. The Law of Attraction maintains that thoughts and emotions emit vibrations that attract similar experiences, whether positive or negative. Ho'oponopono teaches that we are fully responsible for everything that happens in our lives, the result of memories and beliefs that shape our perceptions and decisions. The combination of these practices not only enhances the power of manifestation, but also promotes a deep inner cleansing, essential to open space for abundance, love and personal fulfillment.

When it is understood that limiting beliefs are invisible barriers that block the natural flow of energy, the fundamental role of Ho'oponopono in this process becomes clear. The practice of the four phrases - "I'm sorry. Please forgive me. I love you. I'm grateful." - functions as a purifying agent, dissolving negative memories that feed self-sabotaging thought patterns. Beliefs such as "I am not capable", "I do not deserve to be happy" or "success is not for me" create vibrations that prevent the materialization of dreams. Cleansing these patterns opens space for higher thoughts aligned with the vibration of what you want to attract.

By eliminating emotional and mental blocks, it becomes possible to cultivate positive emotions, such as gratitude, joy and love, which are essential to align personal vibration with the energy of the universe. The Law of Attraction teaches that these emotions function as powerful magnets, attracting situations, people and opportunities that resonate with the same frequency. Ho'oponopono facilitates this alignment by releasing feelings of guilt, fear and anger, allowing energy to flow freely and tune into abundance and fulfillment.

Visualization is another powerful tool that connects these two practices. Imagining with clarity and emotion the achievement of goals sends the universe a clear signal about what you want to manifest. However, for this visualization to be effective, it is necessary to clear doubts and fears that sabotage this process. Ho'oponopono helps to remove these internal barriers, allowing mental images to become clearer and charged with intention. Visualizing goals with confidence and true emotion strengthens the energy vibration, making manifestation more fluid and natural.

However, visualizing and feeling are not enough without action. The materialization of dreams requires concrete steps. The practice of Ho'oponopono promotes the courage and confidence needed to act with determination. By clearing insecurities and fears, the way is opened for more assertive and conscious attitudes. Action aligned with positive thoughts and emotions creates a virtuous cycle of achievement. Each attitude taken with clarity and purpose brings the individual closer to their goals, transforming the manifestation process into something tangible and real.

This integration between thought, emotion and action generates a strong and cohesive vibrational field, ideal for conscious manifestation. It is not about waiting for the universe to deliver results effortlessly, but about acting in harmony with universal energy. This active stance towards life transforms challenges into opportunities, as the individual begins to perceive obstacles as part of the growth process and not as insurmountable barriers. This balance strengthens confidence in the journey and the ability to co-create one's own reality.

Maintaining this practice consistently requires patience and persistence. Manifesting dreams is not an instantaneous process, but a daily construction. Small steps, aligned thoughts and conscious actions build a solid foundation for achievement. The continuous practice of Ho'oponopono ensures that negative memories do not return to block the path, while the Law of Attraction directs energy to materialize desires. This harmony between cleansing the past and creating the future is the secret to a full and fulfilling life.

Furthermore, the integration of these practices stimulates self-knowledge. By identifying and clearing limiting beliefs, the individual begins to better understand their own patterns of behavior and thought. This deep understanding leads to more conscious choices aligned with life purpose. Self-knowledge, in turn, strengthens self-confidence, which is essential to sustain the manifestation process. Knowing who you are and what you want attracts opportunities that are in tune with your true essence.

Over time, this integrated practice transforms not only personal life, but also the way the individual relates to the world. Interpersonal relationships become more harmonious, as personal vibration attracts more authentic and healthy connections. Challenging situations are faced with resilience and wisdom, the result of a clear mind and balanced emotions. Abundance, whether financial, emotional or spiritual, flows more naturally, as there is no longer internal resistance to impede its path.

This transformation extends to all areas of life. In the professional sphere, innovative ideas emerge more easily, and opportunities for growth multiply. In relationships, communication becomes clearer and more empathetic, creating deeper and more truthful bonds. In health, emotional and mental balance is reflected in physical well-being, as body, mind and spirit are aligned. Life as a whole gains more meaning and purpose.

Thus, Ho'oponopono and the Law of Attraction complement each other powerfully. While the former clears the way, removing internal obstacles, the latter directs energy towards the conscious creation of the desired reality. Together, these practices empower the individual to take full responsibility for their life, awakening the unlimited potential to co-create positive and meaningful experiences. From this integration, it becomes possible to live more lightly, authentically and fully, with clarity of purpose and confidence in the flow of life.

Each cleansed thought, each positive emotion and each aligned action forms a bridge between the present and the deepest dreams. This constant connection with the inner essence and with the energy of the universe leads to an existence rich in meaning, love and true achievements. By assuming the role of co-creator of one's own reality, the individual allows oneself to live with more freedom, authenticity and fullness, transforming the journey of life into an extraordinary experience.

By integrating these practices consistently and consciously, each individual begins to recognize the power they have to shape their own reality. The inner purification promoted by Ho'oponopono removes invisible obstacles that limit the natural flow of abundance, while the Law of Attraction directs mental and emotional energy towards the realization of dreams. This harmonious alignment not only transforms challenges into opportunities, but also strengthens confidence in the process of life, allowing the most authentic desires to flourish naturally.

With this new perspective, small daily steps gain meaning, and each choice becomes an opportunity for co-creation. The continuous practice of clearing limiting beliefs, maintaining elevated thoughts and acting with determination builds a solid foundation for lasting achievements. Thus, the journey towards goals ceases to be a path full of obstacles and becomes an enriching experience, guided by purpose, gratitude and inner balance.

In this way, Ho'oponopono and the Law of Attraction are revealed as powerful tools for self-knowledge and manifestation. By uniting these teachings, it becomes possible to live more lightly, consciously and fully. Each cleansed thought, each positive emotion and each aligned action creates a bridge between the present and the deepest dreams, leading to a life rich in meaning, love and true achievements.

# Chapter 33
# Advanced Ho'oponopono

Delving into Ho'oponopono is an essential step to reach higher levels of self-knowledge, healing, and transformation. This advanced stage of the practice transcends the repetition of the four basic phrases and leads to a broader and deeper understanding of the principles that govern this ancestral wisdom. From this expanded perspective, Ho'oponopono becomes an integrated and continuous practice, capable of transforming all aspects of life, promoting balance, inner peace, and harmony in personal relationships and with the world around. It is an invitation to access higher states of consciousness and allow the inner divinity to fully manifest.

At this deeper level, the search for the "zero state" becomes a central goal. This state represents the complete release of memories, judgments, and limiting beliefs, providing a space of silence and mental purity where divine inspiration can flow freely. The connection with the inner divinity strengthens the understanding that we are entirely responsible for our experiences and that we have the power to reframe and transform the reality around us. This recognition expands the awareness that true change begins within each one of us, through the constant purification of thoughts and emotions.

The advanced practice of Ho'oponopono involves the integration of new tools and techniques, such as guided meditations, creative visualizations, and intentional contact with nature and animals. These complementary methods deepen the inner cleansing process and enhance reconciliation with unresolved aspects of life. By applying these practices continuously and consciously, Ho'oponopono ceases to be a punctual action and transforms into a lifestyle, capable of opening paths to a fuller existence, aligned with unconditional love, divine wisdom, and true purpose.

Advanced Ho'oponopono represents a significant deepening in the journey of self-knowledge and healing. This stage goes beyond the repetition of the four fundamental phrases and invites the full integration of its principles into all aspects of life. It is about accessing deeper levels of consciousness, allowing the inner divinity to manifest in an authentic and constant way. In this process, the practitioner understands that true transformation occurs when there is total surrender to the process of cleansing and reconciliation, allowing each experience to be an opportunity for healing.

One of the central concepts at this stage is the "zero state," a state of mental and emotional purity where memories and limiting beliefs are completely dissolved. This inner space, free from interference, is where divine inspiration flows clearly, guiding thoughts, emotions, and actions. Reaching this state means allowing universal wisdom to guide life, without blockages caused by judgments or past experiences. The search for this full emptiness requires constant practice, as each negative thought or emotional resistance represents a new opportunity for purification.

The deep understanding of total responsibility also intensifies in advanced Ho'oponopono. This principle reinforces that everything that manifests in personal reality is a reflection of internal memories, conscious or not. Thus, there is no room for external blame or victimization, but rather for the recognition that each situation is a chance for healing. This acceptance transforms the way of dealing with challenges and conflicts, promoting a more compassionate and loving approach to life.

To sustain this continuous practice, advanced Ho'oponopono integrates complementary techniques that deepen inner cleansing. Guided meditation, for example, allows you to silence the mind and intensify the connection with the inner divinity. During these moments of stillness, the four phrases can be repeated with more depth, accompanied by conscious breathing, allowing the cleansing energy to expand through the body and mind.

Creative visualization is another powerful tool in this phase. By creating clear and detailed mental images of already harmonized situations or achieved goals, the practitioner collaborates with the manifestation process, aligning thoughts and emotions with the vibration of what they want to attract. This exercise, combined with Ho'oponopono, dissolves limiting beliefs and strengthens trust in the natural flow of life, making the realization of dreams more fluid and natural.

Contact with nature also assumes an essential role. Practicing Ho'oponopono in natural environments intensifies the purification process, as the energy of the earth, water, air, and plants facilitates the release of emotional burdens. Walking barefoot on the earth, sitting under a tree, or contemplating the sea while repeating the phrases are ways to deepen the connection with the divine and allow nature to act as an ally in the healing process.

Interaction with animals is another extension of this practice. Animals have a pure and loving energy that can be channeled for emotional healing. Being with them, observing their behaviors, or even directing the Ho'oponopono phrases to strengthen the emotional bond creates an environment of positive energy exchange. This spontaneous and true contact reinforces the importance of simplicity and presence in the present moment.

Integrating Ho'oponopono into every daily action is one of the main pillars of this advanced phase. Each situation, whether simple or complex, can be seen as an opportunity to practice forgiveness, gratitude, and love. Whether facing challenges at work, family conflicts, or feelings of personal dissatisfaction, constant practice allows the mind and heart to stay aligned with inner peace. This continuous integration transforms Ho'oponopono into a lifestyle, where the sacred intertwines with the everyday.

Advanced practice also reveals that personal healing transcends the individual and reverberates in the collective. Each purified memory not only benefits the one who cleanses it but also positively impacts everyone involved in that experience. This awareness expands the purpose of the practice, showing that Ho'oponopono is a tool for global transformation. By healing oneself, one contributes to the harmony of the environment, relationships, and the world as a whole.

This journey requires constancy and surrender, but not perfection. Advanced Ho'oponopono is not based on rigid rules, but on the genuine intention to cleanse, forgive, and love. This daily commitment to purification and inner reconciliation creates a path of lightness and authenticity. Gradually, the practice becomes a silent and constant presence, guiding thoughts, emotions, and attitudes naturally.

Over time, this deep integration generates perceptible transformations. Personal relationships become more harmonious, as the compassionate gaze dissolves judgments and expectations. Challenges are faced with more serenity, understood as opportunities for growth and not as obstacles. The connection with the purpose of life is strengthened, leading to choices more aligned with the true essence. Emotional balance is reflected in physical health, and abundance flows more naturally, without resistance.

Thus, advanced Ho'oponopono presents itself as a path of continuous expansion. It does not promise immediate results, but it offers the opportunity to live in constant evolution. With each cleansed memory, with each purified emotion, the practitioner approaches the zero state, where divine inspiration leads life with lightness and clarity. This state of inner peace does not depend on external circumstances, but is born from alignment with unconditional love and divine wisdom.

This process is an invitation to live with more presence, compassion, and purpose. It is understanding that each cleansed thought, each transformed emotion, and each loving action are steps towards a fuller existence. Advanced Ho'oponopono is not just a technique for individual healing, but a practice of connection with the whole. By assuming this responsibility with love and surrender, we not only transform our reality, but also contribute to the healing of the world.

By deepening this journey, it becomes evident that advanced Ho'oponopono is not limited to isolated techniques, but involves a profound change in perspective on life. Each challenge, each discomfort, comes to be recognized as an opportunity for cleansing and growth. This compassionate gaze allows us to understand that everything that arises on the path is intrinsically linked to the memories we carry, and that, by assuming this responsibility with love and surrender, we open space for true transformation. Thus, the practice expands beyond words, becoming a constant, silent, and powerful presence in every action, thought, and choice.

Over time, this deep integration is reflected in a new way of living, where lightness and authenticity guide relationships and decisions. Advanced

Ho'oponopono teaches that there is no separation between the sacred and the everyday; both are intertwined, and each lived experience carries within it the opportunity for healing. Continuous surrender to the cleansing process does not require perfection, but rather constancy and genuine intention. This openness allows divine wisdom to manifest naturally, leading to a life in balance, where inner peace does not depend on external circumstances, but is born from alignment with the highest purpose.

By walking this path, we understand that Ho'oponopono is not just a practice of self-healing, but a call to awaken the collective consciousness. Each purified memory resonates beyond the individual, positively impacting the environment and the people around them. This understanding expands the purpose of the journey, revealing that by healing oneself, one also contributes to the healing of the world. And so, step by step, the practice unfolds as a continuous flow of love, gratitude, and reconciliation, leading to a fuller existence, harmonious and connected with the divine essence that dwells in each being.

# Chapter 34
# Inspiring Transformation

The personal transformation achieved through Ho'oponopono has the power to expand and positively impact the world around us. By integrating this practice of inner cleansing and reconciliation into your life, it becomes natural to radiate this balance and harmony to other people. This process does not require imposing words or grandiose efforts; it is in the simplicity of daily actions and the authenticity of attitudes that the true impact occurs. Living according to the principles of Ho'oponopono silently inspires those around you to seek their own journey of healing and self-knowledge.

The transmission of this wisdom happens spontaneously when personal experiences and insights are shared with empathy and respect. Whether in intimate conversations or through broader initiatives, such as support groups, social networks, or face-to-face meetings, each gesture of sharing represents an opportunity to sow understanding and peace. By offering Ho'oponopono as a possibility, without impositions, a safe space is created for other people to explore this path freely and authentically. This openness generates deep connections and strengthens the current of collective transformation.

By inspiring transformation in others, the practice of Ho'oponopono itself deepens, consolidating itself as a lifestyle based on responsibility, forgiveness, and unconditional love. This continuous cycle of learning and sharing expands the capacity to generate positive changes, not only on a personal level but also on a collective level. Each conscious action and each word of encouragement contribute to building a more harmonious reality, where individual healing reverberates for the benefit of all humanity. Thus, the practice becomes a link between self-knowledge and the evolution of the world, promoting peace and balance on a large scale.

Sharing the practice of Ho'oponopono is like spreading seeds of light that silently germinate and transform the surrounding environment. When someone genuinely embodies the principles of this ancestral wisdom, the impact is not limited to their own life, but reverberates in all relationships and daily interactions. Without the need for imposing words or great actions, living Ho'oponopono authentically naturally inspires those around us to reflect on their own journeys of self-knowledge and healing. Transformation begins within, but expands to the collective, creating a continuous cycle of love, forgiveness, and reconciliation.

This process of inspiration occurs subtly and spontaneously. The way someone deals with challenges, patience in the face of difficulties, and compassion in relationships become living examples of the practice. Small gestures, such as listening carefully, offering words of support, or acting with kindness, reflect the power of Ho'oponopono in action. This authentic behavior creates an atmosphere of trust, where others feel safe to explore their own emotional blocks and begin a path of healing. It is not about convincing or imposing, but about being a silent example of transformation.

Sharing this practice can also happen through genuine conversations, where personal experiences and learning are transmitted with empathy and respect. Reporting how Ho'oponopono helped to overcome challenges or find inner peace can open doors for others to consider this tool as a possibility in their lives. In intimate settings or wider social circles, this exchange of experiences creates deep connections, nurturing relationships based on understanding and mutual respect. Inspiration, in this context, arises from welcoming and sincere listening, without expectations or judgments.

In addition to personal interactions, sharing can expand to broader platforms. Social networks, for example, are powerful channels for spreading messages of peace and self-healing. Sharing reflections, texts, videos, or even brief accounts of how Ho'oponopono impacts daily life can reach many people seeking tools to deal with their own pain. Creating discussion groups or online communities also promotes safe spaces for exchange, where practices and learning are cultivated collectively, strengthening the chain of transformation.

For those who feel the call to further deepen this sharing, organizing face-to-face meetings, lectures, or workshops offers a rich opportunity for connection.

These moments allow Ho'oponopono to be experienced practically, in a group, enhancing the healing process. Collective experiences, where each participant is invited to explore their emotions and clear limiting memories, strengthen the bond between those present and broaden the understanding of the power of this practice. The environment created in these meetings fosters reflection, self-knowledge, and shared transformation.

Another profound way to disseminate Ho'oponopono is through writing. Producing books, articles, or reflective materials allows knowledge to reach different audiences, contributing to more people having access to this self-healing practice. Recording personal experiences, interpretations of the principles of Ho'oponopono, and suggestions for application in everyday life becomes a valuable gift for those seeking transformation. Writing, like the practice itself, does not have to be perfect, but sincere, fluid, and connected to the purpose of inspiring and welcoming.

However, perhaps the most powerful way to share Ho'oponopono is to live it fully in daily actions. Incorporating forgiveness, gratitude, compassion, and responsibility into every attitude transforms coexistence with others. When these values are practiced consistently, they become part of one's identity and radiate an energy that gently touches everyone around them. Being an example of serenity in the face of conflict, patience in adversity, and empathy in relationships is the purest way to inspire transformation.

This movement of sharing and inspiring strengthens not only others but also the practice itself.

By verbalizing learning or guiding someone on the path of healing, the practitioner deepens their connection with Ho'oponopono and broadens their understanding of internal challenges. This exchange creates a virtuous cycle, where learning is renewed and the responsibility to keep the practice active intensifies. This constant flow of teaching and learning feeds personal evolution and strengthens the connection with the inner divinity.

Inspiring transformation does not require perfection, but presence and intention. It is understanding that every gesture of kindness, every word of comfort, or every positive thought has the potential to trigger significant changes. A sincere smile, attentive listening, or a word of encouragement are silent seeds that bloom in due time. These simple actions, watered by the genuine intention of harmony, expand the reach of Ho'oponopono and invite others to also cultivate inner peace.

This daily and constant practice reinforces the idea that by taking care of oneself, one also takes care of the collective. Each cleansed memory, each transformed emotion, reverberates beyond the individual, creating a more harmonious and balanced environment. This awareness of interconnectedness expands the purpose of the practice, showing that personal healing is not limited to one's own being, but is a silent service to the world. By healing oneself, the practitioner contributes to the healing of the collective, becoming part of a global transformation.

Thus, Ho'oponopono is revealed not only as a practice of self-healing, but as a path to collective evolution. The simplicity and depth of this ancestral wisdom allow it, when lived authentically, to become a silent force for transformation. Each cleansed thought, each welcomed emotion, and each compassionate attitude are threads that weave a network of love and understanding, supporting the construction of a lighter, more harmonious, and conscious world.

In this way, the practice of Ho'oponopono, when lived with truth and shared with generosity, transcends individuality and expands as a collective invitation to healing. It is not necessary to convince or impose; just be, live, and radiate. This is the true power of inspiring transformation: allowing one's own journey to become a light for the path of others, awakening in them the courage to begin their own process of self-knowledge and reconciliation. By inspiring and being inspired, a continuous cycle of love, forgiveness, and evolution is built, leading to a fuller existence aligned with the divine essence.

Sowing peace through Ho'oponopono is understanding that every word, thought, or attitude carries the potential to transform realities. By cultivating compassion and empathy in everyday life, small actions become great gestures of collective healing. A sincere smile, attentive listening, or a simple thought of gratitude can be silent seeds planted in the hearts of those around us. These seeds, watered by the genuine intention of harmony, naturally flourish, inspiring others to also cultivate inner peace and seek their own transformation.

This process does not require perfection, but presence. When we allow ourselves to be vulnerable and authentic, we open space for others to recognize their own humanity and begin their journey of self-knowledge. True inspiration is not in elaborate speeches, but in living with coherence the values we wish to transmit. Thus, the constant practice of Ho'oponopono is reflected in relationships, creating deeper bonds and safe spaces for mutual growth. This shared path strengthens the idea that each one, by healing oneself, contributes to a lighter and more compassionate world.

As each conscious gesture intertwines with the collective, it becomes clear that individual transformation is the first step towards global evolution. Ho'oponopono, lived and shared with love and simplicity, spreads like a breath of light, dispelling the shadows of intolerance and fear. Thus, by sowing peace and healing in ourselves and others, we actively participate in the construction of a more harmonious reality, where love, forgiveness, and responsibility flourish as pillars of a new consciousness.

# Epilogue

Reaching the end of this reading, I realize that it is not an ending, but a new beginning. Each page of this book was an invitation to look inward, recognize one's own shadows, and embrace the light that has always been present. Now, it is up to you to decide the next step.

Ho'oponopono teaches us that true healing does not come from outside, but from the profound act of taking responsibility for everything we experience. With humility, repentance, forgiveness, love, and gratitude, we can dissolve painful memories, restore connections, and allow life to flow more lightly.

May the words "I'm sorry. Please forgive me. I love you. Thank you" resonate in your heart far beyond these pages. May you use them as daily tools for reconciliation with yourself and with the world.

This book was more than an editorial project for me - it was a transformative experience. I hope that, like me, you feel inspired to apply these teachings in every choice, in every silence, in every reconciliation.

Remember: there is no rush. Healing is a continuous and gentle path. Allow yourself to walk with lightness and confidence.

With gratitude for having shared this journey,

www.ingramcontent.com/pod-product-compliance
Lightning Source LLC
LaVergne TN
LVHW041914070526
838199LV00051BA/2615